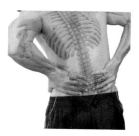
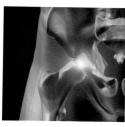
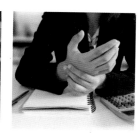

Practical Office
ORTHOPEDICS

Edward (Ted) Parks, MD

Clinical Professor
University of Colorado School of Medicine
Aurora, Colorado

New York   Chicago   San Francisco   Athens   London   Madrid   Mexico City
Milan   New Delhi   Singapore   Sydney   Toronto

Practical Office Orthopedics

5 6 7 8 9 0   DSS   22 21 20

ISBN: 978-1-259-64286-9
MHID: 1-259-64286-0

....

Notice

Medicine is an ever-changing science. As new research and clinical experience broaden our knowledge, changes in treatment and drug therapy are required. The authors and the publisher of this work have checked with sources believed to be reliable in their efforts to provide information that is complete and generally in accord with the standards accepted at the time of publication. However, in view of the possibility of human error or changes in medical sciences, neither the authors nor the publisher nor any other party who has been involved in the preparation or publication of this work warrants that the information contained herein is in every respect accurate or complete, and they disclaim all responsibility for any errors or omissions or for the results obtained from use of the information contained in this work. Readers are encouraged to confirm the information contained herein with other sources. For example and in particular, readers are advised to check the product information sheet included in the package of each drug they plan to administer to be certain that the information contained in this work is accurate and that changes have not been made in the recommended dose or in the contraindications for administration. This recommendation is of particular importance in connection with new or infrequently used drugs.

This book was set in Minion Pro by Cenveo® Publisher Services.
The editors were James Shanahan and Harriet Lebowitz.
The production supervisor was Richard Ruzycka.
Project management was provided by Surbhi Mittal.
The book designer was Eve Siegel.
The cover designer was Randomatrix.

Library of Congress Cataloging-in-Publication Data

Names: Parks, Edward (Edward H.), editor.
Title: Practical office orthopedics / editor, Edward (Ted) Parks.
Description: New York : McGraw-Hill, 2017. | Includes index.
Identifiers: LCCN 2017021245 (print) | LCCN 2017022772 (ebook) | ISBN
   9781259642876 | ISBN 9781259642869
Subjects: | MESH: Musculoskeletal System | Orthopedic Procedures
Classification: LCC RC925.5 (ebook) | LCC RC925.5 (print) | NLM WE 168 | DDC
   616.7—dc23

McGraw-Hill Education books are available at special quantity discounts to use as premiums and sales promotions, or for use in corporate training programs. To contact a representative please visit the Contact Us pages at www.mhprofessional.com.

Contents

Preface

While the health care delivery system in the United States is the subject of much criticism and debate, the medical *education* system in this country is unquestionably among the best in the world. The physicians, physician assistants, and nurse practitioners it produces each year constitute an elite group of health care providers with the knowledge and experience to handle even the most challenging injuries and illnesses. Despite its numerous strengths, one weakness in America's current medical education system is its lack of an adequate orthopedic curriculum for medical students and residents destined for careers in primary care. Many internal medicine residents, for example, feel more comfortable managing a critically ill patient in the intensive care unit than an ankle sprain, and they will see many more ankle sprains, rotator cuff tears, and cases of hip bursitis than they will intensive care unit patients in their practice. In fact, musculoskeletal complaints account for up to a third of the reasons why patients seek evaluation by their primary care providers.

It is this gap in the average medical resident's education that the faculty at the University of Colorado medical center and I sought to fill when we created an outpatient orthopedic rotation for internal medicine residents 20 years ago. The program was well received and very successful. My job was easy: teach orthopedics (perhaps the simplest and most basic of all medical specialties) to some of the brightest minds in health care. Soon, this program and others like it caught the attention of the American College of Physicians (ACP). I began receiving requests to present parts of the curriculum to practicing internists at the regional and, later, national ACP educational meetings. Primary care providers at all stages of their practice careers seemed hungry for this information. In the years since its inception, I have had the opportunity to teach this orthopedic curriculum hundreds of times. Each time, the residents and practicing primary care physicians I work with teach me how to make the presentations better. They help me understand what it is they want to learn and what teaching techniques work best for them.

Practical Office Orthopedics is an effort to put that curriculum together in written form. It is intended to provide the reader with a practical, efficient, and organized approach to outpatient orthopedics and to demystify the practice of musculoskeletal care.

The format of the book is meant to accomplish two very different objectives at the same time. The main text is written to allow quick and easy access to the basic facts. The sidebars in the book emphasize the "backstories" behind some of the conditions presented. The sidebars are written to make the book a more interesting read and, more importantly, to make it easier for the reader to remember the material. As a teacher (and a perpetual student), I am a strong believer in the old axiom: "Hear and I forget. Understand, and I remember." I am also a strong believer in the value of illustrations, so the book is packed with photographs, x-rays, and drawings to help explain the concepts discussed in the text. If this book does its job, reading it should provide you with a practical, easy-to-use approach to the orthopedics you will encounter in a primary care setting.

Ted Parks, MD

Content Reviewers for the American College of Physicians

The following reviewers are gratefully acknowledged:

Suzanne Elizabeth Ames, MD
Associate Professor
Program Director, Orthopedic Residency Program
University of Vermont College of Medicine
Burlington, Vermont

Angela M. Bell, MD, FACP
Internist; Sports Medicine Specialist
Private Practice
Chicago, Illinois

Robert K. Cato, MD, FACP
Chief, Division of General Medicine
Medical Director, Penn Center for Primary Care
Professor of Clinical Medicine
Penn Presbyterian Medical Center
Philadelphia, Pennsylvania

Lisa Miura, MD, FACP
Assistant Professor
Oregon Health and Science University School of
Medicine
General Internal Medicine
VA Portland Health Care System
Portland, Oregon

Balu Natarajan, MD
Private Practice
Chicago Primary Care Sports Medicine
Chicago, Illinois

C. Christopher Smith, MD, FACP
Associate Professor of Medicine
Harvard Medical School
Beth Israel Deaconess Medical Center
Boston, Massachusetts

M. E. Beth Smith, DO
Associate Professor of Medicine
Health Promotion and Sports Medicine
Oregon Health and Science University
Portland, Oregon

Caroline Hines James J. Parks, MD Jim Depuy, MD
gel Roy Meals, MD Mike Lohman Pat Jones Smit
trie Eric Johnson, MD Neil Mackie Tina Ward Willi
ird Pat Bosque, MD Ken Weiner, MD Pete Parks Rom
et Marx Frank Noyes, MD Greg Turner Dow Woodward
oberts Ed Klanecky Chip Larkin, MD Jeff Eckardt, MD
chard David   lard Fillm
Mitchell Pe   rdo Luvig
Laura Lainr   t Marchan
Louise Latir   ow Allen
Miranda Fa   lian Geist
Gerald Mah   is I. Siegel
Carrie Loui   Berenson

THANK YOU!

To my wife, Healy, my children: Shelby, Hudson and Walker, and to everyone else who helped make this book possible

Dave Downs, MD   Mike Carr   Manohar Panjabi Doug Hunley
Allan Moelleken, MD Andy Fine, MD Libby Mauter Bob Eggert
Karen Chacko, MD Paul Elliott, MD Pete Romano, MD   Ted Miclau, MD
David Cromwell, MD David Zimmerman Dan Viders, MD Drew Freeman
Charles Parks Fred Hargadon Jane Parks Ted Warren, MD Patrick Alguire, MD
James C Holmes, MD Fred Teal, MD Ted Clarke, MD Armand Hatzidakis, MD
Raj Bazaz, MD Brian White, MD Tim Birney, MD Tom Mordick, MD Kevin Nagamani, MD
Steve Traina, MD Ben Sears, MD Sean Baran, MD Phil Stull, MD Harriet Lebowitz Phill
James Shanahan McGraw-Hill Publishing Bob Sciortino, MD Susan Valone, MD David Leonard, MD
Mike Gerace Carl Coleman David Hotchkiss Tom Thomas Craig Davis, MD John Belzer, MD Christine
ert W. Sklarew Tony Richie Sam Campbell Ken Easterling, MD Drew Wilson Jeff Reade Matt Comneck
Andrew Waggoner Brian Carter Dan Washburne Ross Goldstein, MD Cameron Bahr, MD   Fernando Boschini, MD
Surbhi Mittal Michelle Andrews, MD Richard Ruzycka Eve Siegel Anthony Landi Jamie Lee Sydne

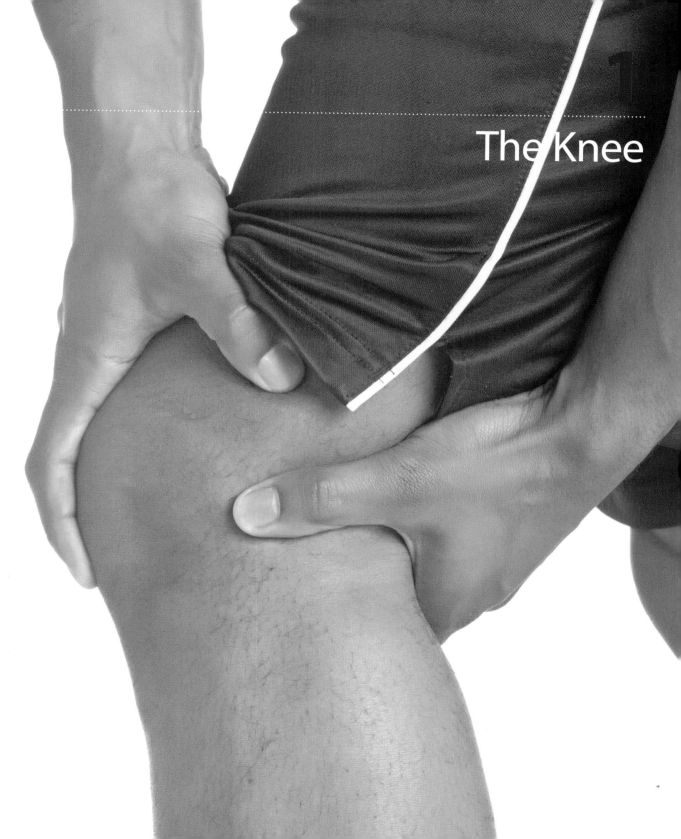

The Knee

THEY ARE NOT CUSHIONS!

I can't tell you how many times I've heard it said that the meniscus cartilages are the "cushions" that reside between the femur and tibia. This isn't true. They do reside between the tibia and femur bones, and it is true that, if a meniscus cartilage is damaged or surgically removed, the articular surfaces adjacent to it will wear out faster. But, the meniscus cartilages are peripheral to the load-bearing contact surfaces in the knee. This deserves a little further explanation. Illustrations like the drawing in Figure 1-4 are misleading. To enable you to see the meniscus cartilages, I have distracted the femur and tibia apart, opening the joint space much wider than it is anatomically. A more accurate representation would be what is illustrated in Figure 1-A. To better understand the relationship between the meniscus, articular cartilage surfaces, and bones, let's study

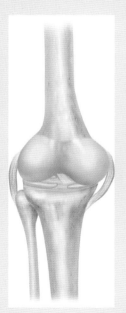

Figure 1-A. A drawing of the knee showing how the meniscus cartilages are hidden from view by the femur.

(continued on following page)

One of the best ways to understand how something, anything, works is to take it apart and put it back together again. For the knee, this is fairly simple. We need a relatively short list of parts: 4 bones, 2 tendons, 4 ligaments, and 2 types of cartilage.

To start, we place the femur, tibia, and fibula bones in their proper positions (Figure 1-1). Next, we need a system of ligaments

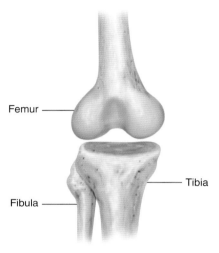

Figure 1-1. Building a knee: the femur, tibia, and fibula bones.

to hold them together (Figure 1-2) and a coating of articular cartilage on the surface of the femur and tibia, two of the three bones that will articulate against each other (Figure 1-3). Of all the structures used to assemble the knee we are building, this thin layer of glistening articular cartilage tissue is probably the most important and the most interesting (please read the sidebar on articular cartilage on page 18). Now we are ready to add the meniscus cartilages, which sit like two rubbery, horseshoe-shaped pads on the surface of the tibia (Figure 1-4). The exact role that the meniscus cartilages play in the function of the knee is poorly understood, but they *do not* act as a "cushion" between the femur and tibia, as many of us were taught (see sidebar). The last bone we need to add if we are building a knee is the patella. The patella is a link in the chain of structures known as the *extensor mechanism* (Figure 1-5). These structures—the quadriceps muscle, the quadriceps tendon, the patella, and the patellar tendon—allow us to forcibly straighten (extend) our knees. When it contracts, the quadriceps muscle (via its quadriceps tendon attachment to the patella) pulls the patella proximally. As it is pulled proximally, the patella (via its patella tendon attachment to the tibia) pulls the anterior tibia proximally, which rotates the knee into extension.

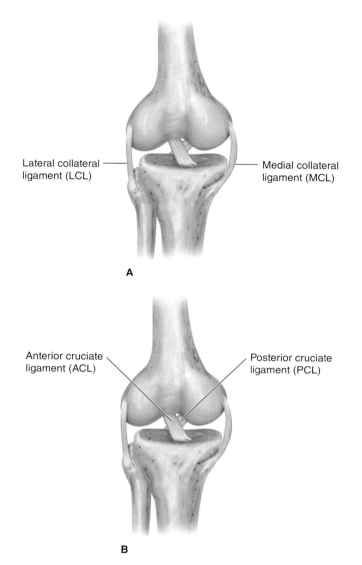

Figure 1-2. **A.** The medial and lateral collateral ligaments. **B.** The anterior and posterior cruciate ligaments.

Having completed the simple "build-a-knee" exercise, it is time to study the different knee conditions seen in a typical outpatient clinic.

LIGAMENT INJURIES

Patients with ligament injuries are usually easy to separate from other patients with knee complaints. The role of the knee cruciate and collateral ligaments is to stabilize the joint. These structures

a series of cross-sectional lateral views (Figure 1-B). Here, we can see that the dimensions and location of the contact patch between the tibia and femur are not affected by the presence or absence of the meniscus. While the exact function of the meniscus cartilages is not known, they do not function as cushions interposed between the articular surfaces of

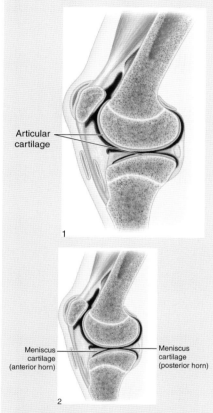

Figure 1-B. A cross-sectional lateral view of the knee **1.** showing the layer of articular cartilage on the surface of the femur and tibia; **2.** showing the anterior and posterior horn of the medial meniscus; **3.** after removing the anterior and posterior horns of the meniscus; **4.** showing the contact patch between the tibia and the femur and how its dimensions are not changed when the meniscus is removed.

(continued on following page)

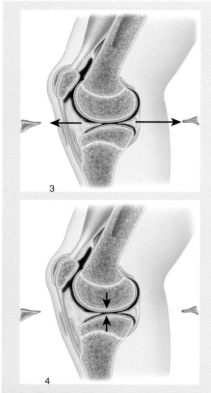

Figure 1-B. (Continued)

the tibia and femur. Figure 1-C shows how this same anatomy appears on a sagittal MRI image of the knee.

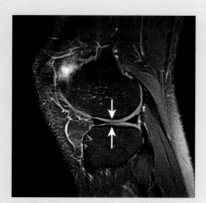

Figure 1-C. How the anatomy in Figure 1-B appears on a corresponding MRI image (Reproduced with permission from Ross Goldstein, MD).

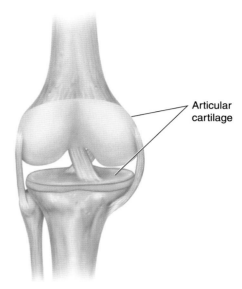

Figure 1-3. The articular cartilage coatings on the surfaces of the femur and tibia.

connect the bones in a way that allows normal motion (flexion and extension) but resists the forces that create abnormal motion (hyperextension; varus/valgus [see further discussion]; anteroposterior translation and rotation). The knee ligaments of

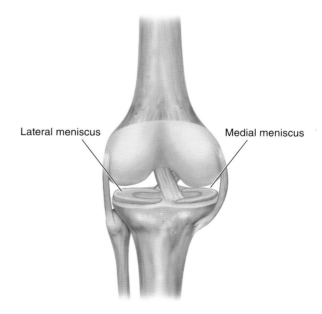

Figure 1-4. The medial and lateral meniscus cartilages.

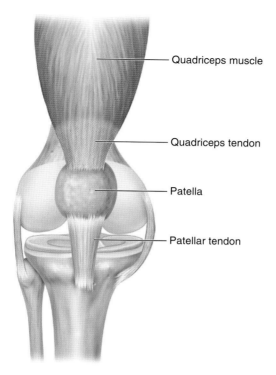

Quadriceps muscle

Quadriceps tendon

Patella

Patellar tendon

Figure 1-5. The extensor mechanism.

a given patient are about the same length and diameter as that patient's pinky finger, so they are essentially impossible to tear without substantial trauma. A patient with knee pain but no history of trauma or injury is not likely to have a ligament injury, at least not a recent ligament injury. You will encounter patients who tell you that they had a "knee sprain" years ago that seemed to heal well, but ever since, they've had a "trick knee" that will give out on them once or twice a year if they twist just right. These episodes of instability are usually followed by a few days to a week of pain and swelling, then the knee returns to normal. This is a classic history for a patient with a chronic ligament-deficient knee. In these patients, the pain and swelling from the initial injury have resolved, but, because the ligament did not heal, they are prone to intermittent episodes of instability. With very few exceptions, trauma, even remote trauma, is requisite in the history for a patient to have a knee ligament injury.

Some patients will offer that they felt, or even heard, a "pop" when the ligament was injured. Knee ligaments are very strong structures. They can store a tremendous amount of energy before failing. If the load is big enough to fail the ligament, then the ligament will rupture, and that stored energy is released suddenly, creating what the patient perceives as a pop. Though not pathognomonic, when patients report a "pop," this important clue strongly suggests a knee ligament injury. An effusion and the timing of its onset can also be important clues, especially when trying to distinguish ligament injuries from meniscal tears. Ligaments are more vascular than meniscal tissue, and patients with ligament injuries tend to develop effusions within an hour of their injury. In patients with meniscus tears, effusions usually develop much more slowly.

▶ Physical Exam

The four knee ligaments, the two collaterals and the two cruciates, each provide a unique and specific aspect of knee stability. Think of the knee as a hinge connecting an upper segment (the femur) to a lower segment (the tibia and fibula). The hinge-like knee joint enables us to flex (bend the knee) and extend (straighten the knee). If the lower segment deviates toward the midline, we call that a varus deformity. If the lower segment deviates away from the midline, we call that a valgus deformity (Figure 1-6). The collateral ligaments are designed to prevent the

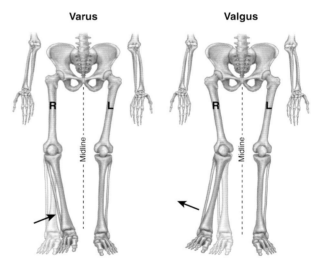

Figure 1-6. Varus and valgus are terms used in orthopedics to describe angular deformities in the coronal plane. In a varus deformity, the distal segment of the articulation (the tibia and fibula in the case of a knee joint) deviates *toward* the midline. In valgus deformities, the distal segment deviates *away from* the midline.

EXAMINING LIGAMENTS

To better understand the knee ligament exam, think of the ligaments as ropes or chains that span the joint like a bridge connecting one bone to the other. The ligaments are positioned not only to allow normal motion but also to resist abnormal motion. When we test a ligament, we apply a force to the knee that attempts to create an abnormal motion and then measure what happens. Specifically, we try to measure two things: the amount of displacement and the quality of the end point. The ligaments are not perfectly rigid; they have a slight amount of elasticity, so they stretch a bit under an applied load. The elasticity of human ligaments varies a great deal from person to person. This helps explain why I have a hard time reaching down to touch my toes, while a contortionist can cross their ankles behind their head. Because of this variability, there is no standard, "normal" amount of displacement to expect when we test a patient's ligaments. The medial side of one patient's knee may open

(continued on following page)

---

lower segment (the tibia and fibula) from swinging back and forth like a pendulum. The medial collateral ligament (MCL) prevents the lower segment from swinging away from the midline creating a *valgus* deformity (Figure 1-7A). The lateral collateral ligament (LCL) prevents the lower segment from swinging toward the midline, creating a *varus* deformity (Figure 1-7B). When the distal segment deviates toward the midline, it is called a *varus* deformity.

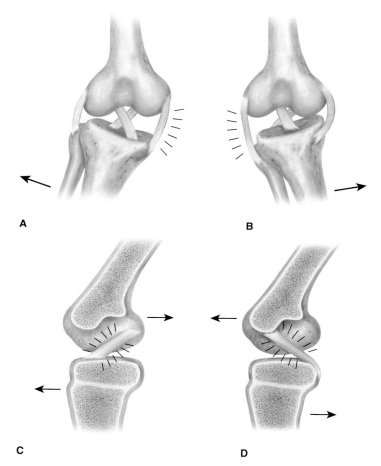

Figure 1-7. A. The medial collateral ligament (MCL) prevents valgus deformities. **B.** The lateral collateral ligament prevents varus deformities. **C.** While the collateral ligaments prevent varus and valgus deformities, the cruciate ligaments prevent anterior and posterior translation of the tibia. The anterior cruciate ligament prevents anterior tibial translation. **D.** The posterior cruciate ligament prevents posterior tibial translation.

Knowing this, we can easily invent the physical exam tests for the collateral ligaments (Figure 1-8). Both tests are done with the patient lying supine, with muscles relaxed and both knees out in full or near-full extension on the exam table. To test the MCL, place one hand on the lower leg and pull it away from the midline while using the other hand to push the thigh toward the midline. Test the LCL by doing the opposite, using one hand to push the lower leg toward the midline while the other hand is pulling the thigh away from the midline. Try to estimate how many millimeters the joint opens and the quality of the "end point" you feel when the ligament stops the knee from moving (see sidebar). If you want to be

2 mm on the MCL test, while another patient's might open a centimeter, and both ligaments could be perfectly normal. To know whether the amount of opening we feel on the ligament exam is normal or abnormal, we have to compare our findings on the knee we are examining to the gold standard: the patient's other, uninjured knee. While there is considerable variability in the elasticity of the ligaments from one person to another, there is little variability when we compare the elasticity of the ligaments of one knee to the other in the same person. A difference of 3 mm or greater between the right and left knees of the same patient suggests a ligament injury.

The "end point" we refer to in the ligament physical exam test is the cessation of motion that occurs during the test when the ligament reaches its elastic limit and displacement stops. In the clinic, I illustrate this to patients by holding my necktie between my two hands. I let it sag a bit, then abruptly tug it tight. The sudden stop that occurs when the tie snaps taut is the end point.

Based on the amount of displacement and the quality of the end point, we can report the findings of the ligament exam using the orthopedic three-grade classification (see Figure 1-9). A grade I ligament injury is one where the ligament is strained, but there is no macroscopic fiber damage. On physical exam, we won't detect any increase in displacement compared to the opposite knee, and there will be a normal, firm end point. The only finding that differentiates a grade I injury from a normal knee on exam is that the patient will experience pain when the ligament is stretched during the test. In a grade II injury, there is a partial tear of the ligament, with some fibers torn and some still intact. In this case, the exam will show increased displacement but a firm end point. In a grade III injury, there is complete rupture of all fibers of the ligament. The ligament exam will demonstrate increased displacement and a soft, mushy end point.

HOW THE ILIOTIBIAL BAND KILLED THE ANTERIOR DRAWER TEST

The ITB is a long, dense, firm band of connective tissue that runs down the side of the thigh. Technically, it is the tendon that connects the gluteus maximus and tensor fascia lata muscles of the pelvis to the lateral side of the tibia just below the knee (Figure 1-D). In the time-honored

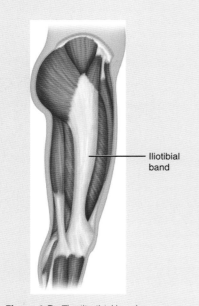

Iliotibial band

Figure 1-D. The iliotibial band.

anterior drawer test, the knee is placed in 90 degrees of flexion, the examiner sits on the patient's foot to stabilize it, and then the examiner pulls the tibia anteriorly to apply a load to the ACL (Figure 1-E).

(continued on following page)

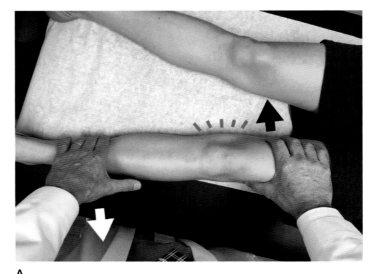

A

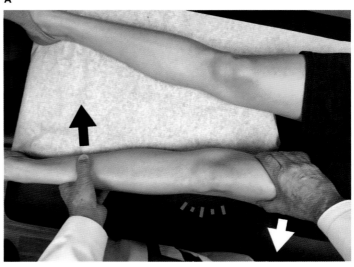

B

Figure 1-8. A. Testing the medial collateral ligament. **B.** Testing the lateral collateral ligament.

fancy, you can use the ligament-grading system described in the sidebar and illustrated in Figure 1-9.

The function of the cruciate ligaments is very different from the function of the collateral ligaments. While the collateral ligaments resist varus/valgus angular deformities in the coronal plane (varus/valgus deformities), the cruciate ligaments resist *translational* motion, specifically anterior and posterior translation of the tibia (Figure 1-7C,D). The examination used to assess the anterior cruciate ligament (ACL) has evolved some in recent years. The

Grading ligament injuries

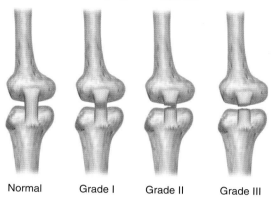

Normal   Grade I   Grade II   Grade III

Figure 1-9. The three grades of ligament injury. In grade I injuries, there is no visable loss of continuity of the ligament tissue, just bleeding/bruising. Grade II injuries are partial tears, and grade III tears are complete tears that result in two un-connected "stumps" of ligament tissue.

anterior drawer test is slowly being replaced by a more accurate test called Lachman's test. In both tests, the examiner tests the ACL by pulling the tibia anteriorly, which pulls the ACL tight; however, what makes Lachman's test superior to the anterior drawer test is that the observed changes in displacement are greater (and therefore easier to detect) using Lachman's test. The reason for the difference is the iliotibial band (ITB), which suppresses anterior tibial translation when the knee is in 90 degrees of flexion (see sidebar).

The *posterior drawer test* is still valid and popular for assessing the posterior cruciate ligament (PCL) because the ITB *shortens* when the tibia is pushed posteriorly (Figure 1-10).

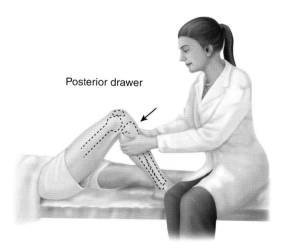

Posterior drawer

Figure 1-10. The posterior drawer test. The knee is placed in 90 degrees of flexion and the tibia is pushed posteriorly.

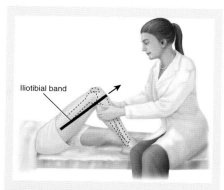

Iliotibial band

Figure 1-E. The location of the ITB in 90 degrees of flexion (the anterior drawer test for a torn ACL).

In 90 degrees of flexion, the ITB is in a position to resist anterior tibial translation, so the amount of translation isn't as obvious. Lachman studied ACL-deficient knees in many different flexion angles and found that the best knee flexion angle for optimizing anterior tibial translation is 30 degrees. In 30 degrees of flexion, the ITB is not in a position to mute anterior tibial translation, so there is greater displacement, which is easier to detect (Figure 1-F).

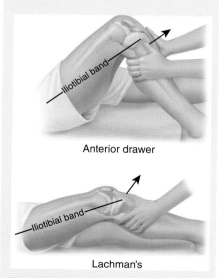

Iliotibial band

Anterior drawer

Iliotibial band

Lachman's

Figure 1-F. Lachman's test for the ACL.

Note that it can be difficult, even impossible due to pain and swelling of the acutely injured knee joint, to perform a meaningful ligament exam on an acutely injured knee. If the patient is too uncomfortable to relax for the exam, the options are to repeat the exam in 1-2 weeks when the pain has decreased or to obtain a magnetic resonance image (MRI).

▶ *Imaging Studies*

If the mechanism of injury is trauma, which it usually is for knee ligament injuries, x-rays are probably warranted to rule out a fracture. This trauma may be contact trauma (i.e., two football players colliding) or noncontact trauma (a soccer player running down the field makes a cutting move and twists his or her knee). Anytime there is a history of significant trauma, an x-ray should be taken to rule out a fracture. Another imaging option is an MRI. An MRI is a very specific and sensitive test for evaluating ligament injuries, and it will pick up fractures as well. For suspected ligament injuries, the MRI can help diagnose patients who are too uncomfortable to be examined acutely or too impatient to be reexamined a week or two later to confirm the diagnosis on physical exam.

▶ *Medical (Nonoperative) Treatment*

The cruciate and collateral ligaments live in very different physical environments. The collateral ligaments are extra-articular. They are surrounded by vascular soft tissue and have blood vessels inserting along their entire length to nourish them. As a result, nearly all collateral ligament injuries, even grade III injuries (complete, full-thickness tears resulting in two, unconnected ligament "stumps"), heal well without surgery. Treatment goals are to optimize patient comfort, minimize atrophy and stiffness, and support the injured ligament as it heals. A brief period (2 weeks) on crutches and in a knee-immobilizing brace (Figure 1-11) followed by motion and strengthening exercises is a typical recommendation. Transition to a hinged brace (Figure 1-12) at 2 weeks may be necessary for high-grade injuries; low-grade injuries can transition from the straight leg brace to no brace at all.

Cruciate ligaments live in an environment that is very different from that of the collateral ligaments. They have a relatively poor blood supply, spanning the joint space with no blood vessels inserting along their length. For this reason, complete, full-thickness cruciate ligament injuries do not heal. The fate of partial cruciate ligament tears depends on how much ligament tissue is still intact. For example, those with more than 90% still intact do well, those with less than 10% intact are likely to fail at some point in active patients. While it is possible to differentiate partial (grade II) tears from complete (grade III) tears on the physical

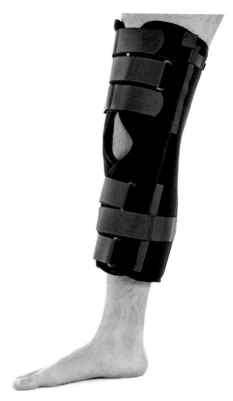

Figure 1-11. The straight leg knee immobilizer brace. This brace is rigid and does not allow any type of knee motion *(Licensed from Shutterstock)*.

exam (see the sidebar in this chapter on examining ligaments), it is impossible to use the physical exam to determine exactly how much of the ligament remains intact in partial tears. Some have advocated obtaining an MRI on suspected partial tears so that those with high-grade partial tears can be identified and considered for surgical treatment.

▶ Surgical Treatment

Grade III (complete) cruciate ligament injuries (and the rare grade III collateral ligament injuries that *don't* heal) result in ligament-deficient knees. In general, ligament-deficient knees are not well tolerated by patients and require surgical reconstruction. As mentioned, collateral ligament injuries, even complete tears, typically heal without surgery. The few torn collateral ligaments that don't heal can often be successfully repaired (their torn ends sutured back together) or reconstructed with a graft. Because of their poor blood supply, torn *cruciate* ligaments will not heal with suture repair and have to be replaced with a graft. Grafts can be

THE THEORY OF "THE NEUROMUSCULARLY ELITE"

The dogma as it relates to ligament-deficient knees, specifically ACL-deficient knees, is that ligament deficiency results in arthritis. While this is true in many, perhaps even most, patients, it is not true for *all* patients. An ACL-deficient knee will usually have a specific pattern of instability: In certain sports or activities, the knee will experience a force that tries to drive the tibia anteriorly with respect to the femur above it. Without an ACL to counteract this force, the tibia slides farther forward

(continued on following page)

than it should, allowing the condyles of the femur to strike the posterior horns of the meniscus cartilages. This results in meniscus tears, and meniscus tears accelerate the rate of wear of the knee's articular surfaces, which in turn results in arthritis. But, patients who are sedentary are unlikely to apply the knee stresses necessary to create instability. A simple and brief course of muscle strengthening in physical therapy can give them the stability they require for the modest demands of daily activities. These patients can do well treated nonoperatively. What's interesting is that there are a few humans out there who aren't sedentary, who can still be quite active on their ligament-deficient knees *without experiencing any instability!* (Figure 1-G) Although it is controversial, one explanation is that

ACL tears ⟶ Arthritis

ACL tears → Instability → Meniscus tears → Arthritis

ACL tears ⇸ Instability → Meniscus tears → Arthritis

Figure 1-G. The relationships between ACL deficiency and the development of arthritis. The accepted fact is that ACL tears result in arthritis. This is because, in most patients, ACL tear result in a pattern of instability that creates meniscus tears, which leads to arthritis. For some patients, ACL tears do not result in instability, so they don't get arthritis.

these patients have a better proprioceptive system than the rest of us, and, when the tibia starts to translate too far anteriorly, they fire a compensatory hamstring muscle contraction that arrests the pathologic motion of the tibia. Best estimates are that these individuals account for less than 5% of the population, and, as of right now, we don't have any reliable way to test for this gift. For now, the consensus recommendation favors ACL reconstruction in active patients because 95% of them will experience a pattern of instability that eventually results in arthritis.

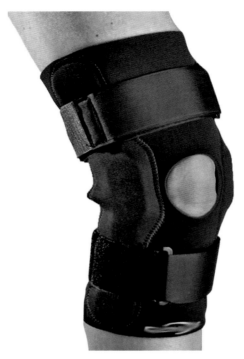

Figure 1-12. The hinged knee brace. There are hinges built into the medial and lateral sides of this brace that allow flexion/extension, but not varus/valgus or hyperextension.

either from the patient's own tissue (autograft) or from cadaveric donors (allograft). Artificial (synthetic) grafts and grafts from nonhuman animals have been tried and have not worked well.

Recovery after ACL surgery is long, 6-12 months, but results are generally very good, with high rates of return to sports and strenuous activities. Keep in mind that not all ligament-deficient knees require surgery. The goals of ligament reconstruction surgery are a) to eliminate symptoms of joint instability and b) to help prevent the pattern of arthritis that these patients typically experience *years or decades* after their injury. Rarely, patients with ligament-deficient knees *do not have instability* (see sidebar, page 11). Patients who don't have instability do not need surgical reconstruction to stabilize their knees … or do they? This is somewhat controversial. There is a body of evidence that suggests that some of these patients who have no subjective sense of instability have a pattern of "micromotion" instability that, over the course of decades, results in destructive arthritis. If this is true, then the only ACL-deficient patients who should be treated nonoperatively are those who both (a) have no instability symptoms and (b) are old enough that, for these patients, the development of arthritis 20 or 30 years down the road is inconsequential.

MENISCUS TEARS

Figure 1-4 shows what the meniscus cartilages look like as they sit on the articular surface of the tibia in the knee joint. These thin, rubbery tissues can tear, and when they do, they can be a source of knee pain. Figure 1-13 shows what a typical meniscus tear looks

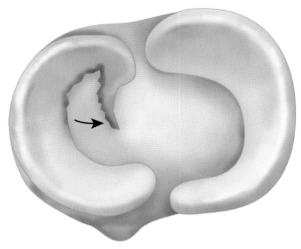

Figure 1-13. A torn meniscus.

like when we view the meniscus cartilages from above. The history that patients with meniscus tears give is unique in that their chief complaint is pain at the joint line, medially or laterally. In young patients, the meniscus is tough and durable, and it is hard for a person under the age of 25 to tear their meniscus without some element of knee trauma. Usually, this is a weight-bearing, twisting injury. As we age, the meniscus cartilage becomes more fragile. In patients over age 50, it is possible to tear the meniscus cartilage by simply squatting. In the squatting position, the prominent posterior part of the femoral condyle (see discussion that follows) bears down hard and pinches the meniscus between the femur and tibia. Add a little twist, and you might just end up with a torn meniscus. Some patients with meniscus tears will experience catching or locking or other mechanical symptoms as the piece of torn meniscus flips intermittently in and out of the joint.

▶ *Physical Exam*

The three best tests for detecting a meniscus tear are joint line tenderness, pain at the joint line with deep flexion, and McMurray's test. To test for joint line tenderness, we must first identify the location of the joint line. To find the joint line, have the patient lie supine on the exam table with their knee flexed 90 degrees. Find the patella anteriorly. On either side of the very inferior part of the patella, there is a soft spot. This soft spot is the anterior joint line (it opens when the knee is flexed). Follow the joint line around medially and laterally all the way back to the back of the knee. Most meniscus tears are in the posterior part of the meniscus, so don't forget to go all the way back posteriorly. Tenderness to palpation at the joint line medially or laterally may indicate that your patient has a meniscus tear.

The deep flexion test takes advantage of the fact that the end of the femur isn't round; it is oblong, or "cam" shaped, with an extra lobe of bone protruding posteriorly (Figure 1-14). This extra

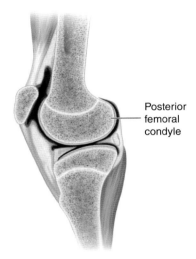

Posterior femoral condyle

Figure 1-14. The posterior femoral condyle.

lobe of posterior femur bone bears down on the meniscus in deep flexion. If the meniscus is torn, pinching it like this between the femur and tibia in the deep flexed position is likely to re-create the patient's pain (the deep flexion test).

McMurray's test is very hard to describe without physically demonstrating it on a knee or knee model. The maneuver is a combination of knee flexion, rotation, and angular (varus/valgus) stress. To test the medial meniscus, have the patient lie supine with the lower extremity to be tested flexed 90 degrees at the hip and knee (Figure 1-15). Grasp the patient's foot with one hand and their knee with the other. Externally rotate the hip joint as far as it will go (this will bring the foot and leg across the midline). *Note: do not perform this test on patients with a hip replacement. It can cause dislocation.* Now, rotate the tibia by rotating the foot while flexing and extending the knee. The first step (hip rotation) closes the medial joint and pinches the medial meniscus between the tibia and femur. The second step (rotation/flexion-extension) "grinds" the meniscus between the two bones, which will cause medial joint line pain in most patients with a medial meniscus tear. McMurray's

▶ *Physical Exam*

High mileage may be the only reliable feature in the patient's history to indicate osteoarthritis, and pathognomonic physical exam findings are equally scarce. Joint swelling, stiffness, tenderness to palpation, and even warmth may all be present, but again, they are not specific to the diagnosis of arthritis. The one physical exam finding that is very specific for knee joint arthritis is the presence of severe angular deformities (Figure 1-17). Mild angular

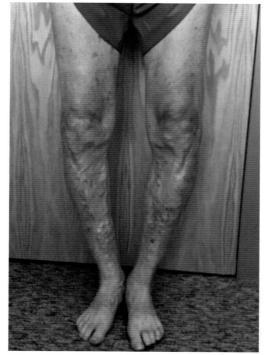

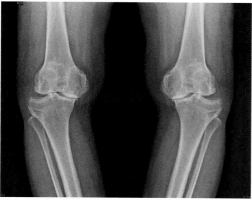

A

Figure 1-17. **A.** Medial wear creates a varus (bowlegged) deformity.

essentially a bearing surface and, as such, has several unique properties and characteristics. For one, it is incredibly slick and slippery. Lubricated with the thick, viscous synovial fluid in the joint, articular cartilage bearing against articular cartilage has a coefficient of friction better that that of an ice skate on ice! It is much more slick and slippery than anything we have been able to invent to take its place. This unique mechanical property allows us to move our joints easily and smoothly. Articular cartilage has a unique biological property as well: It has no sensory innervation. It has no nerves in it and no capacity to feel touch, pressure, impact, or friction. This is an important feature because our joint-bearing surfaces are under significant loads and stresses as we use our bodies every day. Unfortunately, in addition to the attributes of slickness and numbness, articular cartilage has another, less helpful, feature that makes it unique when compared to other types of tissue. It has no capacity to heal or regenerate. As a result, the articular surfaces in all of our joints wear with daily use and the passage of time. There are a few conditions that can hasten the wear rate of articular cartilage. An intra-articular infection can, in hours or days, destroy a layer of cartilage that would otherwise take a lifetime to wear away naturally. Injuries that directly damage the articular cartilage can cause post-traumatic arthritis, and injuries that result in bone deformities that alter the loads on our joints can overload discrete patches of the articular surface and create focal areas of rapid wear. There are a handful of rheumatologic conditions in which chronic intra-articular inflammation destroys the articular cartilage. Rheumatoid arthritis is one such disease. In patients with a strong family history of arthritis, we often see inherited subtle skeletal deformities that load joints abnormally. Or, a softer, less durable cartilage may be passed on in a particular family lineage. Repetitive

(continued on following page)

trauma from work or sports can certainly accelerate the rate of cartilage wear. No matter how you get there, arthritis is the term we use to describe the state of cartilage loss on the articular surface of a joint. This loss of the articular cartilage bearing surface has grave consequences. It turns out that just below the thin, glistening layer of slick, numb articular cartilage is the worst bearing surface you could imagine: bone. Bone is not slick and slippery; it is rough and abrasive, and it is loaded with sensory nerves (if you've ever had your teeth worked on, you know how sensitive bone is). The end stage in arthritis is "bone-on-bone" arthritis, where the rough, sensitive surface of one bone grinds against the rough, sensitive surface of the other bone in the joint. As you would predict, this creates a stiff, painful joint, and it explains the symptoms that our arthritic patients have. Fortunately, most of us will live out our lifetimes without wearing through the articular cartilage surface down to bone. But, if the science of medicine is ever successful in keeping us all alive for 200 years, one of the problems we will face is the unavoidable loss of articular cartilage down to bone that would occur over that period of time.

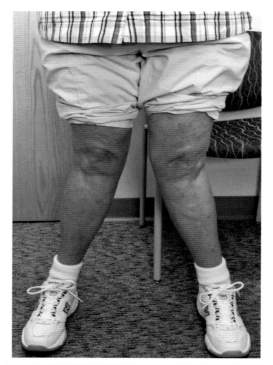

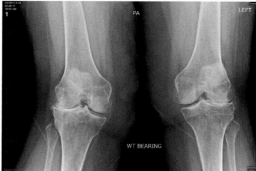

B

Figure 1-17. (*Continued*) **B.** Lateral wear creates a valgus (knock-knee) deformity.

deformities can exist in normal knees, but severe deformities usually indicate the presence of arthritis. In third world countries, severe angular deformities can result from nutritional deficiencies (rickets), but in developed countries, these angular deformities are almost certainly associated with asymmetric, down-to-bone patterns of articular surface wear. Medial joint wear results in varus (bowlegged) deformities, and lateral-sided wear results in valgus (knock-knee) deformities. These wear patterns and their resultant deformities can be unilateral or bilateral.

A quick-and-easy office physical exam screening tool is to have the patient lie supine on the exam table and ask them to squeeze their legs together. If the anatomy is normal, their ankles and knees will touch at about the same time. If they have medial wear on one or both knees, the ankles will touch first (bowlegged/varus deformity). If they have lateral wear, their knees will touch first (knock-knee/ valgus deformity). Again, mild varus and valgus angular deformities can be considered normal, but severe deformities likely indicate arthritis.

▶ *Imaging Studies*

For the diagnosis of arthritis, there is no single clinical tool that is more useful than a properly taken set of x-rays, and there is no clinical tool as useless as an improperly taken set of x-rays. For this reason, let's spend a moment reviewing how we go about getting the views that will help us the most. First, we have to avoid ordering a "knee series." At most facilities, this order will get you a non–weight-bearing AP, a lateral, and a pair of oblique views. This series was designed for evaluating patients in the emergency room, where injured patients can't weight bear and have limited range of motion. This emergency room series is well suited for looking for fractures but is a poor choice for the evaluation of an office patient in whom we suspect arthritis. A better set of x-rays to order is as follows:

1. **A weight-bearing AP view** (Figure 1-18). In Figure 1-18, the knee on our left is normal, with relatively well-preserved articular cartilage. The knee on our right has bone-on-bone medial arthritis. The difference in the space between the bones is very clear on this weight-bearing AP x-ray. We are going to use this

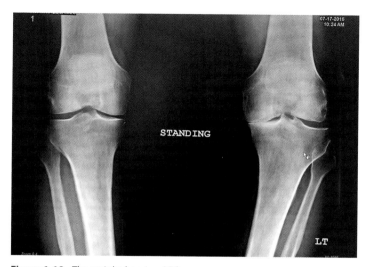

Figure 1-18. The weight-bearing AP knee x-ray.

view to evaluate the thickness of the clear space between the tibia and femur. That space is narrowed or completely absent if they have significant arthritis. But, even a patient with bone-on-bone arthritis may *appear* to have a decent space between the tibia and femur if a non–weight-bearing x-ray is taken because the surfaces of the two bones relax away from each other. *A non–weight-bearing AP x-ray can make a closed (bone-on-bone) joint space look open.* We need the weight-bearing force to press the two surfaces together. Figure 1-19 shows the technique used to shoot a proper weight bearing AP x-ray of the knee.

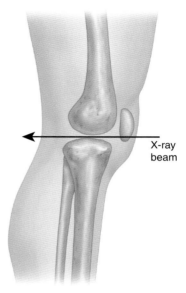

X-ray
beam

Figure 1-19. Taking a proper weight-bearing AP knee x-ray. To obtain this view, the patient has to be standing with their knees extended (straight) and fully weight bearing on both lower extremities. The radiology technician must direct the beam parallel to the floor and exactly at the level of the joint. Assessing the space accurately also requires that the x-ray beam is truly parallel to the top surface of the tibia. You can only appreciate the open space between two flat, parallel surfaces if your line of sight is parallel to those surfaces. Look down from above, or up from below, and the space disappears. *An off-axis x-ray can make an open joint space look closed.*

2. **A weight-bearing, flexed knee, posterior-anterior (PA) view** (Figure 1-20). This view, also called the Rosenberg view or a weight-bearing notch view, can detect a very common pattern of knee arthritis that would otherwise be hard to detect. Imagine a patient who has lost all of the articular cartilage on the surface of the tibia and on the posterior part of the femur. If this patient still has a layer of articular cartilage on the anterior part of the femur, they will still

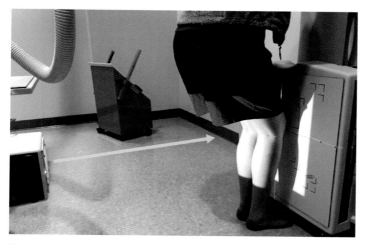

Figure 1-20. Taking a proper weight-bearing PA flexed knee x-ray.

have a space between the tibia and femur on the weight-bearing AP x-ray (which is taken with their knee extended). If we take a weight-bearing *flexed* knee view, flexing the knee rotates the "bald spot" on the posterior femur to be opposite the bare area on the tibia, resulting in an x-ray that shows bone-on-bone contact between the tibia and femur (Figure 1-21). X-rays of a patient with this pattern of arthritis are shown in Figure 1-22. The image on the left in

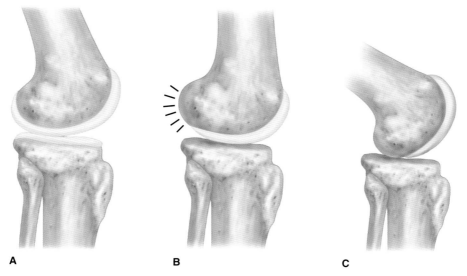

A   B   C

Figure 1-21. A. A knee with normal articular cartilage surfaces weight bearing in extension. **B.** A knee in the same position, but with complete loss of tibial cartilage and loss of the cartilage on the tibia and posterior part of the femur. **C.** The knee shown in B in the weight-bearing flexed knee position.

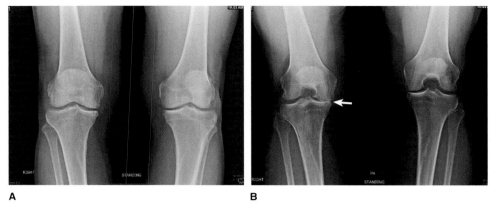

A

B

Figure 1-22. The same knee x-rayed using the weight-bearing AP technique (**A**) and the weight-bearing flexed knee PA technique (**B**). Note the area of bone-on-bone wear visable on the flexed knee view (arrow) that is not visable on the view taken with the knee extended.

Figure 1-22 is a weight-bearing x-ray of an arthritic knee with the knee in the extended position. This view is taken as an AP image, with the film directly behind the knee and the x-ray beam shot from the front. The photo on our right shows the same knee imaged using the 60-degree PA weight-bearing view technique, revealing bone-on-bone arthritis on the medial side of the knee. It is taken with the knee flexed, but the x-ray beam is still parallel to the top surface of the tibia (Figure 1-23). The intracondylar notch

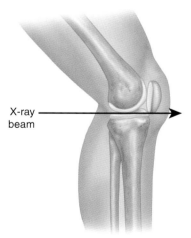

X-ray beam

Figure 1-23. How to position the patient and the x-ray beam for a flexed knee weight-bearing PA view. It is difficult to put the film flat against the back of the knee in this view because the knee is bent, so the film is placed in front of the knee, and the x-ray beam is shot from posterior to anterior. Care must be taken when shooting this view to keep the x-ray beam parallel to the surface of the tibia, which may not be parallel to the floor when the knee is bent.

between the two condyles of the femur is much easier to see in the flexed knee view than the extended knee view, so this view is sometimes known as the *weight-bearing notch view*.

3. **A Merchant view (also known as a sunrise view or sub-patellar view).** While the loss of articular cartilage on the surfaces of the tibia and femur results in the most common pattern of knee arthritis, wear between the patella and the anterior femur can also be a source of arthritic pain. To detect wear in this part of the knee joint, we need to "peer" under the knee cap. This can be done by placing the patient, the film, and the x-ray beam as shown in Figure 1-24. A normal

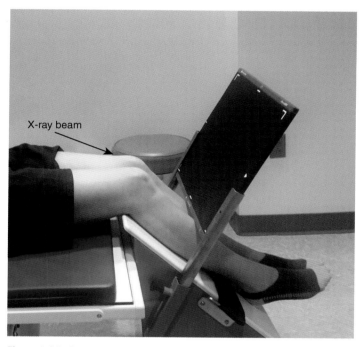

Figure 1-24. Positioning a patient for a Merchant view x-ray.

Merchant view x-ray is shown in Figure 1-25. An x-ray showing bone-on-bone patella-femoral arthritis is shown in Figure 1-26. Patella-femoral arthritis is part of the spectrum of patella-femoral syndrome, discussed further in this chapter. Patella-femoral pain syndrome, including patella-femoral arthritis, is often bilateral and more common in women than in men; symptoms typically include anterior location of pain and pain that increases with descending stairs, squatting, and prolonged sitting.

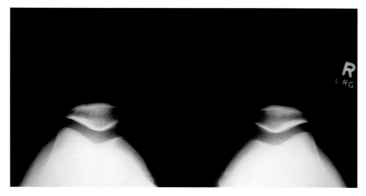

Figure 1-25. A normal patella-femoral joint as seen on the Merchant view x-ray, also known as the sunrise or subpatellar view.

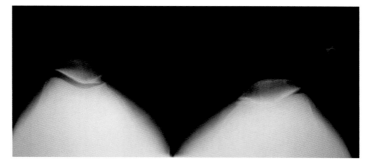

Figure 1-26. Bone-on-bone arthritis of the patella-femoral joint as seen on the Merchant view x-ray.

4. **A lateral view.** The flexion angle and weight bearing versus non–weight bearing are not important here. Of all the x-ray views, this view gives us the least helpful information.

Requesting (and receiving) the proper x-ray views makes a big difference when it comes to diagnosing knee arthritis. Know the facility where your patients are getting their films and let the facility know what views you need. Otherwise, you are likely going to receive the standard knee series views, and you will be missing out on one of the simplest, most cost-effective and accurate tools used in the diagnosis of knee arthritis. If possible, view the films yourself, and, when practical, share them with your patients. The analysis is quick and simple, and the sight of bone-on-bone arthritis on a knee x-ray is a visual demonstration that explains the patient's problem to them in a way that almost every one of them will understand.

▶ Medical Treatment

In many cases, knee arthritis, even bone-on-bone knee arthritis, can be treated nonoperatively. There appear to be two sources of pain in the arthritic knee. One results from the direct stimulation of the exposed nerve endings on raw bone surfaces (again, think of the dentist touching a cavity with a metal probe). The other may come from the pressure that a joint effusion creates inside the joint (see sidebar). NSAIDs, either prescription or over the counter, help by deflating the swollen joint and taking pressure off of the capsule. Unfortunately, NSAIDs aren't always safe for these patients. They are ideal for the 24-year-old with a sprained ankle. That patient will likely have excellent renal function and will only need the medication for the few weeks it takes for the ankle to heal. Patients with arthritis tend to be older and more medically frail. It is often necessary for patients with arthritis to take high doses of NSAIDs for long periods of time, perhaps indefinitely, and we know that high doses of NSAIDs over long periods of time in medically frail patients can lead to serious gastrointestinal (GI) and renal complications. For this reason, a cortisone shot may actually be safer and more effective treatment for knee arthritis than oral anti-inflammatory medications. It provides better joint pressure decompression than NSAIDs, and it is without the attendant GI and renal side effects. (Please refer to Chapter 9 for instructions on how to administer a safe and simple knee cortisone injection.) Other conservative treatment options include the following:

A. **Viscosupplementation injections.** These are injections of high-molecular-weight polymers of hyaluronic acid. We know that hyaluronates are an important constituent of healthy synovial fluid, and these thick, viscous injections may help with joint lubrication. If there is a beneficial effect to these injections, it is subtle. Several well-designed studies have failed to demonstrate statistically significant results. Despite relatively flimsy supporting evidence, these injections were able to secure Food and Drug Administration approval for the treatment of osteoarthritis, and some patients with arthritis do appear to respond to them. Contrary to the claims of some manufacturers, they have not been shown to add cartilage or any other protective substance to the surface of arthritic joints.

B. **Oral supplements** (see sidebar, page 28).

C. **Braces.** There are several types of braces designed for the treatment of injured and arthritic knees. The most basic is the straight leg knee-immobilizing brace (see Figure 1-11). This brace is intended to eliminate knee motion and is better suited for treating injured knees than arthritic knees. For acute exacerbations of chronic arthritis, one could potentially make a case for a brief period in an immobilizing brace, but using

---

THE BLISTER ON YOUR TOE COMES FROM THE PEBBLE IN YOUR SHOE

Arthritis is a productive process. We've all seen older people with arthritic knuckles: The joints are huge! Arthritis produces extra material that increases the size of the joint. It produces extra bone (osteophytes or bone spurs), extra tissue (synovial hypertrophy), and extra joint fluid (the arthritic effusion). It is known that the rough articular surfaces in an arthritic joint create more friction as they rub against each other, creating a signal that the joint needs more thick, viscous lubrication fluid. The excess joint fluid in an arthritic joint appears to be the body's attempt to better lubricate the failing joint. Anything that irritates the inside of the joint—a torn meniscus, a small volume of blood (blood is a potent inflammatory agent), or the rough surface created by the partial or complete loss of articular cartilage—will create an effusion that stretches the joint capsule. The stretching pressure on a joint capsule overstuffed with synovial fluid contributes to the pain and stiffness typical of an arthritic joint. In the knee, that joint capsule, which extends circumferentially 360 degrees around the joint, is weakest posteriorly. If the pressure is great enough for a long enough period of time, the patient can develop a swollen "bulge" posteriorly where a bubble of fluid-filled joint capsule herniates out into the soft tissue between the hamstring tendons. This posterior collection of displaced joint fluid is known as a Baker's cyst. Many patients will discover these cysts and become quite concerned. They can be a source of pain, and some patients will ask that they be drained or removed. Unfortunately, draining, or even surgically removing, the Baker's cyst doesn't tend to work, at least not for long. The cyst typically returns because the stimulus for

(continued on following page)

the overproduction of joint fluid remains in the joint. The treatment that is most effective at ridding patients of their Baker's cyst is whatever treatment will address and eliminate the intra-articular irritation. This can be an operation, a cortisone injection, or, perhaps, a viscosupplementation injection. Once the source of inflammation is addressed, the Baker's cyst will subside. If you have a blister on your toe, draining or removing the blister is not likely to work. A better solution is to remove the pebble from your shoe. Once you do this, the blister will resolve on its own.

GET ME TO A BARBER SHOP ... STAT!

Most of the oral supplements recommended for knee arthritis (glucosamine sulfate, chondroitin sulfate, MSM, SAM-E, hyaluronate, etc.) are chemicals that are found in articular cartilage. The thought is that if articular cartilage is what is missing, then taking large volumes of the ingredients that constitute articular cartilage should help it regenerate. Unfortunately, our bodies don't work that way. If they did, I would drop what I am doing right now, run to the nearest barber shop, and eat all of the hair off of the floor so that I could fill in this nasty bald patch I have on the top of my head!

The fact is that no oral or injected medicine has ever been shown to add articular cartilage to the surface of an arthritic joint. Despite that fact, many patients report improvement of their arthritic symptoms after taking these joint supplements. In some studies, the degree of improvement exceeds what one would expect from the placebo affect alone. It may be that these supplements are working to decrease pain, but the mechanism of their action has yet

(continued on following page)

this brace to treat arthritis is unusual. Hinged braces, which allow flexion and extension but prevent hyperextension, varus, valgus, and other abnormal motion patterns, are also known as ligament substitution braces (see Figure 1-12). Their medial and lateral hinges can substitute for or support injured ligaments, and because ligament dysfunction isn't the issue in knee arthritis, the use of these braces for this condition is not evidence based. The same can be said of the use of neoprene sleeve braces. These thin, flexible, pull-on braces may keep the joint warm and heighten proprioceptive feedback, but they do not alter the mechanics of an arthritic joint in any significant way. One brace designed specifically for the treatment of knee arthritis is the "unloading" brace. This brace only works for patient's whose arthritis is confined to one side (medial or lateral) of their knee. For patients with medial-side arthritis, for example, the brace is intended to apply forces to the knee that move the distal tibia laterally, shifting the joint's articular surface contact forces away from the worn, sensitive medial side of the joint and onto the less affected lateral side of the joint (Figure 1-27). Unloading braces can be worn full time, or just for strenuous activities, and it does appear that they may work for some patients. Unfortunately, the benefit of the unloading brace is gone as soon as the brace is removed.

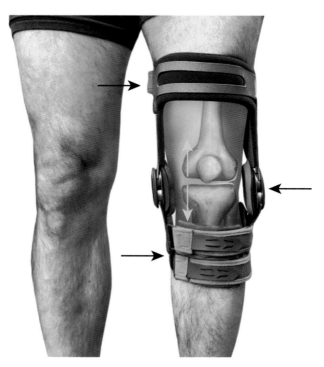

Figure 1-27. An unloading brace for medial knee joint arthritis.

D. **Weight loss.** Reducing knee joint compressive forces by losing weight can decrease the pain of arthritis. Weight loss is difficult for any patient, but even more difficult for patients with knee pain due to arthritis. A weight loss program for these patients must rely heavily on dietary restrictions, and some limited, low-impact exercises like swimming or biking.

E. **Assistive devices (cane, crutches, walker).** As is true with weight loss, using these devices reduces knee joint compressive forces and can decrease pain.

F. **Physical therapy and exercise.** One might predict that the effect of exercises that involve repeated knee motion under load might be to *increase* the symptoms of arthritis, and for many patients, this is true. Numerous studies, however, do support the notion that, for patients who can tolerate them, low-impact, non–weight-bearing exercises and physical therapy can help alleviate the discomfort of knee arthritis. This observation may result from the effect that physical therapy and motion have on increasing joint capsule flexibility and compliance, which could decrease pain by allowing the joint capsule to distend more easily, thereby lowering intra-articular pressures due to swelling.

G. **Other ideas.** The preceding list of nonoperative treatment options for knee arthritis is by no means exhaustive. It represents what most practitioners would consider "standard" conservative treatment options. If a personal favorite of yours is not outlined here, please don't be offended. There are many other remedies (some orthodox, some unorthodox) that have been tried with some success (see sidebar).

▶ Surgical Treatment

Several interesting operations have been used to address the problem of knee arthritis in the past (see sidebar, page 30), but modern surgical solutions all aim to "re-pave" the damaged joint surfaces with a new coating of slick, slippery, numb, and durable material. We use metal and high density polyethylene plastic to replace the bearing surface of articular cartilage. Most patients misunderstand what is done in a knee replacement operation. The name *total knee replacement* implies that we are going to cut across the femur somewhere above the joint and cut across the tibia somewhere below the joint and replace the entire joint. This conception isn't accurate. What we do is more like what a dentist does when a cap is applied to a tooth. We do cut a small amount off of the very surface of the tibia and femur, and then we bond a "cap" of metal and plastic to the ends of the bones to take the place of the lost articular surface cartilage. A better name for the procedure would be a total knee *surface* replacement. A total knee replacement refers to an operation that resurfaces the entire tibia and femur. A partial

to be elucidated. After all, in the history of pharmaceuticals, there have been many instances where a beneficial effect is observed years or decades before the mechanism of action is discovered.

THE LATEST AND GREATEST: VOODOO, SNAKE OIL, THE PLACEBO EFFECT, AND WHAT JUST MIGHT BE THE NEXT BIG THING WE'LL ALL BE USING IN FIVE YEARS

Surface magnets, laser light treatments, stem cell injections, platelet rich-plasma injections, copper bands, topical creams, acupuncture—the list goes on and on. Do these things work? Should we be using them for our patients? Do we have an obligation to limit our treatment recommendations to those that are evidence based and supported by the rigors of randomized, prospective, double-blinded, statistically significant studies? How much of our job is art, and how much is science? There probably isn't any one correct answer to these questions, but the strategy I think works best and is most ethical is to remember that, as physicians, we are essentially scientists, and any good scientist is, by nature and by necessity, a skeptic. If you are scientist, being a skeptic is part of your job description. We owe it to our patients to carefully and scientifically vet the flood of good and bad information that they encounter on their quest for a solution to their medical problems. In my opinion, this means not only *recommending* proven treatments, but also discussing unproven treatments. Stick with what is known and proven, but at the same time, realize that our science is often inexact. If we dogmatically close our eyes to all new, unproven, or unorthodox treatments, we may miss out on the benefits

(continued on following page)

of treatments and techniques that later prove to be what's best for our patients. Sure, being a skeptic is an important part of being a good scientist, but so is maintaining an open mind when it comes to entertaining new and unconventional ideas.

A COUPLE OF CRUMMY OPERATIONS

Before the 1960s, the surgical solutions to knee arthritis left a lot to be desired. One popular operation was the knee arthrodesis, or "knee fusion" (Figure 1-K).

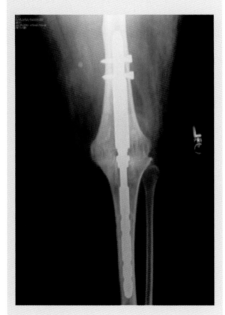

Figure 1-K. A knee joint arthrodesis (fusion).

In this procedure, the distal end of the femur and the proximal end of the tibia are removed with a saw. The raw, exposed bone surfaces of the tibia and femur are then approximated with a rod or a set of plates and screws. Held in rigid apposition

(continued on following page)

knee replacement (or unicompartmental replacement) refers to an operation where only part (the medial tibia and medial femur, for instance) of the knee is resurfaced. The patella can also be resurfaced by bonding a plastic dome to the part of it that articulates with the femur.

Knee replacement surgery has led to a substantial decrease in pain and significant improvement in quality of life for hundreds of thousands of patients each year since the operation was introduced decades ago. If a patient with bone-on-bone arthritis has pain that is limiting their activities and they have failed conservative management, a knee replacement is often a great solution. Other, less common, indications include severe varus or valgus deformities or advanced erosive changes on x-ray. Postoperative complications such as infection, stiffness, and continued pain spoil the results in a small number of patients, and we are still trying to perfect a knee replacement that is guaranteed to last a lifetime for all patients (see sidebar, page 36).

There is no question that a better surgical solution to the problem of knee arthritis would be a biological resurfacing technique. It may be that stem cell or other technology will someday enable us to apply a new layer of living cartilage to arthritic joints, and this would be far superior to resurfacing them with metal and plastic as we do today. Imagine the thrill you would feel as an archeologist coming across one of these metal and plastic total knee replacement devices a million years from now. You would instantly know that the layer of dirt that you are working in is from sometime between 1960 and 2040 when humans used this primitive technique of applying metal and plastic to the ends of each other's bones!

PROBLEMS OF THE PATELLA-FEMORAL JOINT

Patella-femoral knee pain is often referred to as "the low back pain of the knee." It is extremely common, and our treatments don't work all that well. This makes patella-femoral pain a frustrating topic for physicians and patients. The "classic" elements in a patient's patella-femoral syndrome history are listed next. Take a mental photograph of Figure 1-28. If you see this patient (a female with anterior knee pain, worse with descending stairs), chances are you are looking at a patient with patella-femoral pain.

The classic symptoms of patella-femoral syndrome are as follows:

A. **Female gender.** This condition is much more common in women than in men (see sidebar, page 38).

B. **Bilaterality.** The anatomic factors that predispose one knee to this condition are likely present on the opposite knee as well.

C. **The pain is usually anterior: on, under, or around the patella.**

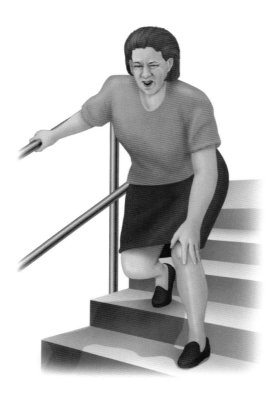

Figure 1-28. The classic example of a patient whose knee pain is coming from the patella-femoral joint: a woman with anterior knee pain (often bilateral) that is worse when descending stairs.

D. **The pain is usually worse with stairs (especially descending stairs), worse with squatting, and worse with prolonged sitting (the "theater sign").** Any activity that applies a compression force to a flexed knee is likely to exacerbate patella-femoral pain.

▶ Physical Exam

The relevant physical exam findings for patella-femoral syndrome can be boiled down to three categories:

A. **Patella-femoral joint mobility.** The mobility we are interested in is medial-lateral mobility; to test for it, have the patient lie supine on the exam table with their knees extended and their muscles relaxed. Gently move the patella medially and laterally (Figure 1-29). A normal patella should move between 25% and 75% of its own diameter. Excessive motion suggests patella-femoral instability. Less than 25% mobility suggests a stiff, arthritic joint.

B. **Gross patellar mal-tracking.** With the patient seated on the edge of the exam table, ask the patient to flex and extend their knee a few times. In patients with gross patella-femoral

like this, the two surfaces of bone will grow together like the two surfaces of a fractured bone do when they are immobilized next to one and other. The result is one solid bone that extends from the hip to the ankle. The pain of the worn ends of the femur and the tibia grating against each other inside of the knee is gone, but at a price: The knee joint is permanently frozen in the extended position. This seemingly barbaric operation was one of the early surgical solutions to knee arthritis. The fact that most patients who had this operation preferred it to the pain they had prior to surgery demonstrates how severe and disabling the pain from knee arthritis can be. The other operation we could offer arthritic patients before the 1960s was an osteotomy (Figure 1-L).

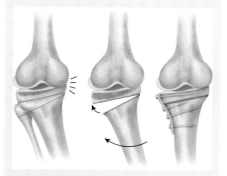

Figure 1-L. The high tibial osteotomy (HTO) operation for medial or lateral arthritis (example shown is for medial arthritis).

This procedure, which is essentially the surgical version of the unloading brace (see main text), was designed to help patients with wear that was isolated to the medial or lateral side of the joint. Figure 1-L shows a joint with down-to-bone wear in the medial compartment (left drawing). The middle drawing shows the first part of the operation, which is to remove a pie-shaped slice of the tibia, creating a triangular gap in the bone that

(continued on following page)

is closed as the shaft of the tibia is rotated laterally. The last part of the operation (drawing on the right of Figure 1-L) is to rigidly lock the two parts of the tibia back together so that they can heal in this new position. The end result is to shift the tibia laterally and transfer weight-bearing loads from the deteriorated medial side of the knee to the relatively healthy lateral side (or vice versa, for lateral-side arthritis). The obvious advantage of this operation over a knee fusion is that motion is preserved. The downside to the procedure is that the pain from bone-on-bone articulation isn't eliminated, only diminished. There is still bone-on-bone contact on the affected side on the joint, but it is under less compressive force, so the pain it generates is less severe.

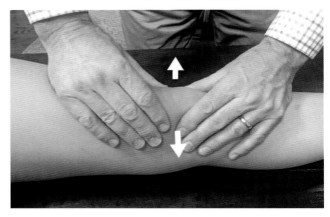

Figure 1-29. Checking patella-femoral joint mobility.

mal-tracking, the examiner can see the patella jump in or out of the femoral sulcus as the knee passes through a flexion/extension range-of-motion cycle.

C. **Crepitation.** Repeat the exam in part B with the palm of your hand on the patient's patella. Alternatively, you can flex and extend the patient's knee for them with your hand on their patella (Figure 1-30). The crunching, grating, or grinding you

FILLING POTHOLES

Articular surface wear (arthritis) can result in large areas of cartilage thinning or having down-to-bone change. The cartilage loss in arthritis is likely to be on both sides of the joint, specifically, in the areas where the articular surfaces of the two bones bear against each other. The weight-bearing knee x-ray on the right in Figure 1-18 shows such a pattern of down-to-bone articular cartilage loss on both the medial femur and medial tibia of an arthritic knee. A very different type of articular cartilage loss can result from trauma. In the case of traumatic loss, articular surface cartilage isn't worn away slowly over years or decades, but "chipped off" suddenly by a traumatic blow. The area of cartilage loss is usually smaller, with sharp, discrete edges, and these lesions are usually isolated to the surface of just one bone. Figure 1-M shows a dime-size area on the surface of the femur where the articular cartilage has been knocked off traumatically, resulting

(continued on following page)

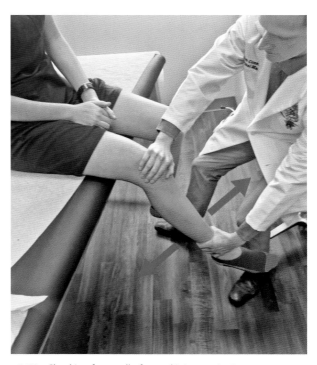

Figure 1-30. Checking for patella-femoral joint crepitation.

feel is crepitation in the patella-femoral joint. Many asymptomatic patients have this crepitation, so it is only significant when it is disproportionately severe on the symptomatic knee, in which case it may signify advanced patella-femoral joint articular cartilage wear.

▶ Imaging Studies

The Merchant view x-ray (discussed previously) is the simplest and most cost-effective imaging tool we have for evaluating the patella-femoral joint. Figures 1-25 and 1-26 show Merchant view x-rays of normal and arthritic knees. Figure 1-31 shows a Merchant view

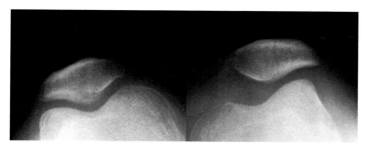

Figure 1-31. A Merchant view x-ray showing normal (left) and abnormal (right) patellar tracking.

x-ray demonstrating patellar mal-tracking. Figure 1-32 shows an example of combined mal-tracking and bone-on-bone arthritis,

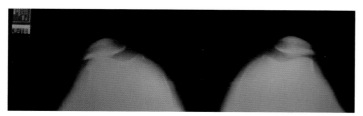

Figure 1-32. A Merchant view x-ray showing combined patella-femoral arthritis and patellar mal-tracking.

and Figure 1-33 shows severe, end-stage, bone-on-bone arthritis with erosive changes on the patellae and femur.

▶ Medical Treatment

Patella-femoral syndrome can be difficult to treat. Physical therapy combined with a short treatment of NSAIDs can help. The therapy exercises are intended to strengthen the medial quadriceps and loosen the lateral retinaculum to facilitate better patellar tracking. Several types of braces exist for this condition as well. The most common is a simple pull-on sleeve brace with a hole

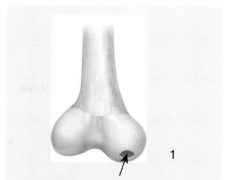

Figure 1-M. A dime-size area of traumatic cartilage loss.

in an area of exposed bone. The articular cartilage surrounding this area of injury is healthy and normal. We have developed several surgical procedures to try to restore or replace small areas of traumatic cartilage loss like this one. None of them work particularly well, with success rates hovering around 70%, and none of these techniques is well suited for the treatment of the cartilage loss seen in arthritis, where the regions of exposed bone are larger, on both surfaces of the joint, and lack distinct, healthy cartilage borders.

TECHNIQUE 1: WHAT IS A "MICROFRACTURE," AND WHY WOULD I EVER WANT ONE?

The microfracture technique (Figure 1-N) is an attempt to create a fibrocartilage plug to fill the pothole defect. The name is confusing because it is neither microscopic nor a fracture. In this technique, which is usually done arthroscopically, a tool shaped like an ice pick is used to make several deep perforations in the bone at the base of the pothole defect. These small-diameter holes allow blood from deep within the bone to weep onto the exposed surface and organize into a clot that forms a fibrous patch to fill the defect. This fibrocartilaginous patch does not have the mechanical or biological

(continued on following page)

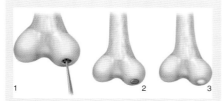

Figure 1-N. The microfracture technique: The bone at the base of the defect is perforated multiple times with a tool that resembles an ice pick (**1**). Blood from deep in the bone weeps out through these perforations and forms a clot over the defect (**2**), which matures into a layer of fibrocartilage (**3**).

properties of articular cartilage (it is not as slick or durable, and it usually has some degree of sensory innervation), but it is better that an untreated area of raw, exposed bone.

TECHNIQUE 2: HAIR PLUGS, ANYONE?

The osteochondral (bone and cartilage) autograft (graft from the patient) transfer/transplant surgery (also known as the "OATS procedure"; Figure 1-O) takes

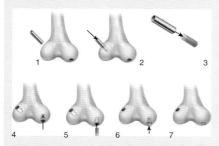

Figure 1-O. The OATS technique: A steel tube is used to harvest a dowel-shaped plug of bone and cartilage from an area where the articular cartilage does not articulate (**1-3**). A drill is used to convert the defect into a deep tunnel (**4**), and the graft is inserted into the tunnel (**5-7**).

(continued on following page)

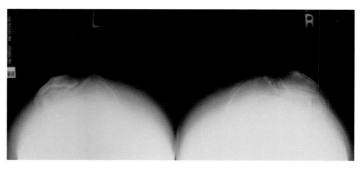

Figure 1-33. A Merchant view x-ray showing advanced bone-on-bone arthritis of the patella-femoral joint in both knees with bone loss due to erosive changes.

in the front to help center the patella (Figure 1-34). These braces may help correct mild cases of patellar mal-tracking. There is a more complicated, less common brace that uses springs to assist eccentric quadriceps contraction (see sidebar, page 36).

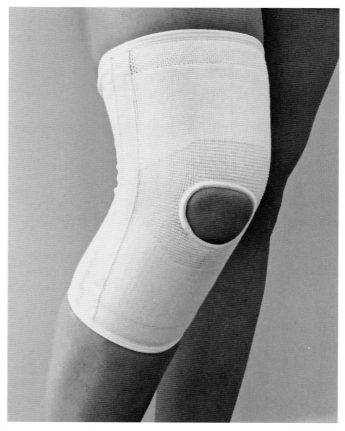

Figure 1-34. A patella-femoral sleeve brace.

Eccentric quadriceps contraction occurs when we apply a load to a bent knee and our quadriceps extension force is used to counterbalance the knee flexion force created by gravity. Patella-femoral compression forces are high during eccentric quadriceps contraction, and decreasing the magnitude of the quadriceps eccentric contraction force by adding external spring support has been shown to be effective in decreasing patella-femoral compression force.

A cortisone injection can help here as well. Inflammation in the patella-femoral joint can lead to swollen synovial lining tissue, which can become pinched in between the bones in the joint. As is the case when you bite the inside of your cheek, the more swollen the tissue is, the more it tends to be pinched, and the more it is pinched, the more swollen it becomes. This can set up a self-perpetuating cycle, and a cortisone injection can break that cycle. (See Chapter 9 to learn a simple, effective knee injection technique.)

▶ Surgical Treatment

Many of the surgical procedures designed to address patella-femoral syndrome have had relatively poor results in terms of patient satisfaction. A major challenge is that this part of the knee seems to be particularly sensitive to even small amounts of articular cartilage loss or irregularity. The operations we have to correct patellar mal-tracking are unable to reverse articular surface wear, so while the operation may be successful in slowing the rate of wear by correcting patellar tracking, the irritation from thinning articular surface wear is not improved. The arthroscopic lateral release (Figure 1-35) attempts to correct patellar mal-tracking

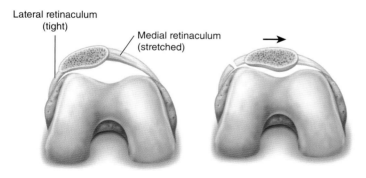

Figure 1-35. Releasing the lateral patella-femoral retinaculum to improve patellar mal-tracking.

by loosening the lateral retinaculum. Some surgeons will combine this technique with an imbrication of the medial soft tissues, while others believe that tightening any part of the patella-femoral joint should be avoided because it could increase contact forces. A medial patella-femoral ligament (MPFL) reconstruction can help stabilize patellae prone to lateral tracking, as can a tibial tubercle

advantage of the fact that there are several small areas on the surface of the femur that are coated with articular cartilage and do not articulate with the tibia or patella. Cartilage is harvested from one of these areas by tapping a 3- to 10-mm diameter (depending on the size of the graft that is needed to fill the defect) steel straw deep into the femur bone to remove a dowel-shaped "plug" of bone with a cartilage cap. Then, a drill is used on the area of articular surface loss to create a tunnel into which the plug graft is inserted. The base of the graft will heal bone to bone with the bone in the tunnel, securing the cartilage cap into place on the articular surface. The procedure is similar to a popular hair transplant technique, where plugs of hair are transferred from the nape of the neck to the front of the scalp.

TECHNIQUE 3: HOME GROWN

This third technique involves two separate surgical procedures (Figure 1-P). In the first procedure, an arthroscope is used to harvest a small sample of articular cartilage from an area on the surface of the femur that does not articulate with

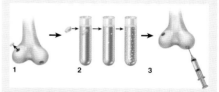

Figure 1-P. The autologous chondrocyte transfer technique: A small sample of articular cartilage is harvested arthroscopically from an area of the femur that does not articulate with either the patella or the tibia (**1**). The sample is sent to a lab, where the extracellular matrix is removed, and the cells are grown in tissue culture (**2**). A patch of periosteum is sewn over the defect, and the chondrocytes are injected under this membrane, where they secrete a matrix to heal the defect with a new layer of articular cartilage (**3**).

(continued on following page)

the tibia or patella. This articular cartilage sample is then sent to a lab, where the extracellular matrix is removed and the chondrocytes are allowed to grow and multiply for 8-10 weeks in tissue culture. In a second operation, the knee joint is exposed via an open incision and a thin membrane of periosteum is sewn over the chondral defect like a drum skin. The cultured chondrocytes are injected under this periosteal membrane and into the articular surface defect. Some of the cultured chondrocytes survive and secrete new matrix material, filling the pothole with fresh articular cartilage.

HOW LONG DO THEY LAST?

A major challenge in joint replacement surgery is to design an operation that yields a lifelong result for all patients. It is not unreasonable to expect a modern total knee replacement in a patient over 60 years of age to last their lifetime. Patients between 50 and 60 should probably expect at least one revision in their lifetime, and patients who are younger than age 50 at the time of their initial replacement may require so many revision operations that they fail and become unrevisable before the patients die. The most common mode of failure for knee replacements is aseptic loosening. Just like a cap on a tooth will eventually come loose and fall off, the bond between the knee replacement components and the bone eventually fails and the components become loose. The patient perceives this looseness as pain as the loose part shifts and moves against the sensitive bone beneath it. On x-ray, we see it as a lucent line between the knee replacement component and the bone. Several factors are thought to

(continued on following page)

transfer, in which the angle of patellar tracking is changed by surgically moving the insertion of the patellar tendon medially (Figure 1-36). It is important to keep in mind that any operation

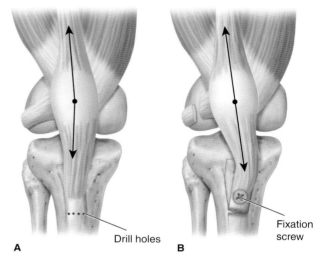

A   B

Figure 1-36. The tibial tubercle transfer operation.

in which the tissues around the patella-femoral joint are manipulated in any way can result in an imbalance in the strength of the four members of the quadriceps muscle, which can be detrimental to patella-femoral joint function and adversely affect the surgical outcome. The surgical treatments outlined are only considered when patients have exhausted extensive nonoperative management and continue to suffer from symptoms they cannot tolerate. The success rates of these operations are not as good as they are for most other knee surgeries.

OTHER KNEE CONDITIONS YOU WILL ENCOUNTER

The conditions detailed previously cover the most common knee problems that you are likely to see in an outpatient office setting. If your patient's signs and symptoms don't seem to match any of these, he or she may have one of the periarticular conditions listed next.

A. **Pes anserine (pes) tendonitis.** The tendons of three thigh muscles, the gracilis, the sartorius, and the semitendinosus, all insert together on the medial part of the proximal tibia, just inferior to the joint line (Figure 1-37). Early anatomists thought that these three tendons looked like a *pes anserinus* (Latin for the "foot of a goose"). The name stuck. Patients can develop an insertional tendonitis here if one or more

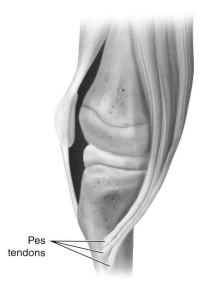

Pes
tendons

Figure 1-37. The pes tendons on the anteromedial tibia inferior to the medial joint line.

of these tendon attachments becomes inflamed. This has come to be known as pes tendonitis. There is also a bursa between the tibia bone and these tendons, which, when inflamed, results in a pes bursitis. It is almost impossible to differentiate pes tendonitis from pes bursitis clinically, but the treatment is the same, so it may not matter. Patients with pes tendonitis/bursitis will complain of anteromedial knee pain *below the joint line* and, on physical examination, will be tender to palpation of the anteromedial tibia *below the joint line*. Treatment for both conditions is ice, rest, NSAIDs, and physical therapy. The physical therapy program for pes tendonitis/bursitis involves hamstring and groin muscle stretches and eccentric (see sidebar, page 40) exercises and can include modalities such as ultrasound and iontophoresis (a topical application of corticosteroid and low-energy electric current). If these fail, a cortisone injection at the pes insertion onto the anterior-medial tibia can help. A simple technique for administering a pes tendonitis/bursitis cortisone injection is presented in Chapter 9.

B. **Iliotibial band insertional tendonitis.** The ITB (see sidebar Figure 1-D) is a long, slender tendon that connects the gluteus maximus and tensor fascia lata muscles of the pelvis to the lateral tibia. It inserts onto the lateral side of the proximal tibia just below (distal to) the knee joint. It is sort of the "mirror image" of the pes tendons. Patients can develop an insertional tendonitis of the ITB at its insertion onto the

affect how long these bone/component bonds last.

A. **The quality of the initial surgery.** If the components are installed in improper alignment and abnormal loads are applied to the bone/component interface, the longevity of component fixation will be adversely affected.

B. **Activity.** Active patients apply more force more frequently to their total knees. Over time, these forces, especially the impact of running on hard surfaces, is thought to hasten the failure of the bone/component bond.

C. **Age.** It has long been observed that knee replacements in younger patients fail sooner than knee replacements in older patients. Initially, it was thought that this observation was a reflection of the difference in activity between older and younger patients. While it is true that, on average, younger patients are more active than older patients, there is more at play here than just age-related differences in activity. If you control the activity level of younger patients to match that of older patients, the replacements of the younger patients *still* fail sooner. The younger patients are at a biological disadvantage. To understand this disadvantage, imagine you spill superglue onto your hand. After a few days, the glue finally comes off, not because the glue failed, but because the skin cells that the glue was bonded to die and are replaced by new cells that are not bonded to the glue. This same process of cell turnover occurs in bone. It doesn't occur in days, like skin, but in years or decades. Bone turnover rates are much faster in young patients and they slow down significantly as we age. This accelerated bone turnover rate is the biological factor that shortens the longevity of knee replacements in young patients, and it is independent of activity.

THE CURSE OF THE Q

As the knee passes through its normal extension and flexion range of motion, the patella glides up and down in a shallow groove, called the femoral sulcus, on the anterior surface of the femur (Figure 1-Q).

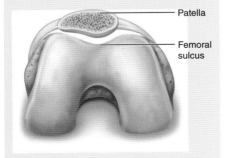

Figure 1-Q. The patella articulating with the femoral sulcus of the femur.

The contact forces, which can be several multiples of body weight in activities such as descending stairs and squatting, are born by the thin layer of articular cartilage that coats the articulating surfaces of these two bones. If the patella is tracking in the center of the femoral sulcus, then these forces are shared over a relatively large surface area. If patellar tracking is off by even a few millimeters (Figure 1-R), then those same forces are borne by a relatively small patch of

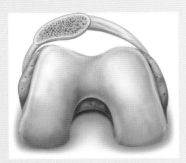

Figure 1-R. A mal-tracking patella.

(continued on following page)

proximal lateral tibia. These patients will complain of pain on the lateral side of the knee joint that is *below the joint line*. On physical exam, they will be tender to palpation on the lateral side of the tibia *below the joint line*. Pain and tenderness at the lateral joint line are more consistent with a lateral meniscus tear. As is the case with pes tendonitis/bursitis, the recommended treatment is rest, ice, NSAIDs, and physical therapy, specifically (you guessed it) gluteal, ITB, and tensor fascia lata stretches and eccentric strengthening exercises. One can also give a cortisone injection at the site of tendon insertion onto the lateral tibia or at the spot where the ITB rubs against the lateral femoral condyle, if that is where the pain is.

C. **Patellar/quadriceps tendonitis.** Tendonitis of the extensor mechanism tendons (the quadriceps and patellar tendons; see Figure 1-5) typically occurs where the tendons attach to bone. Patients with quadriceps and patellar tendonitis will have patella-femoral symptoms (anterior knee pain that is worse with descending stairs, squatting, lunges, and prolonged sitting). But, they will lack significant asymmetric crepitation on knee flexion/extension and will be point tender over the superior pole of the patella (quadriceps insertional tendonitis), the inferior pole of the patella (proximal insertional tendonitis of the patellar tendon), or the tibial tubercle (distal insertional tendonitis of the patellar tendon). They may have pain at these locations when you test resisted knee extension (have them sit on the edge of the exam table with their knee out in extension, then ask them to push against you while you try to flex their knee. This recruits all members of the extensor mechanism). Treatment is once again rest, ice, NSAIDs, and a physical therapy program that emphasizes extensor mechanism stretches and eccentric progressive resistance exercises. Cortisone injections are not recommended into or near the patellar or quadriceps tendons due to an associated increased risk of tendon rupture.

▶ WHAT IF YOU ARE STILL STUMPED?

No matter how complete your knowledge of knee conditions is and no matter how experienced you are at diagnosing and treating orthopedic patients, you will encounter patients whose knee problem makes no sense to you. The inability to make a diagnosis in these patients does not in any way reflect a deficit in education or competence; it is just one of the cold, hard facts of patient care in the real world that some knee problems elude our diagnostic tools. I see several of these patients in my practice *every day*. Many cases don't fit the diagnosis and treatment patterns we were taught in the classroom, on the wards, or in textbooks like this one. Because these "diagnosis unknown" cases are so common, we need to have a strategy that helps us deal with them in a practical, safe, and cost-effective way. Here is the approach I use:

A. **Rule out other "non-knee" pathology.** Many patients with hip and back problems present with a chief complaint of knee pain. Identify patients whose knee pain comes from a radiculopathy by asking for symptoms such as pain that shoots down from their hip to their toes; electrical, shooting pains in the same distribution; and numbness and tingling in their ipsilateral foot and toes. On physical exam, these patients may have specific patterns of weakness, sensory loss, or diminished deep tendon reflexes (see Chapter 6, page 181, for details). Along with radiculopathies, hip pathology is famous for presenting as knee pain. A great screening test is the "windshield wiper test." For details on this physical exam test, check out Chapter 3, pages 90 and 91. A simple, inexpensive AP pelvis x-ray can help, too. I can't tell you how many times in the over 25 years that I have been doing this that I have come across a patient with knee pain who has a completely normal knee (and no complaints of hip pain!) but has an arthritic hip, radiating pain down to their knee.

B. **If you can't explain their pain based on a lumbosacral radiculopathy or hip joint pathology, you may have to accept the fact that you simply have no idea what's going on with the knee of this particular patient.** And, it is possible you never will. While I've always believed my grandmother when she taught me that honesty is the best policy, disclosing to a patient that you haven't a clue what's wrong with them never seems to go over well. Instead, I tell them that I am very confident that all of the important structures in their painful knee—the ligaments, tendons, bones, and cartilages—are all strong and healthy. I recommend three things:

1. Two weeks of over-the-counter ibuprofen (600 mg three times a day with food, provided there are no GI, renal, or other contraindications).
2. Simple home stretches: Stretch the hamstrings by standing bent at the waist and reaching down to try to touch your toes; stretch the quadriceps by standing and pulling the heel to the buttock, one leg at a time. I ask that they hold each stretch for 30 seconds to a minute, 10 times a day.
3. Ride a stationary bike 20 minutes a day, 5 days a week.

They are asked do this program for 1 month. They are instructed that if they are not better after a month, they are to return to the office, and, if they do come back, I choose ONE of the following:

1. **I order physical therapy.** I write a very general prescription: gait training, weight bearing as tolerated, progressive resistance exercises, stretches, and, if the therapist feels they are indicated, modalities like therapeutic ultrasound, iontophoresis, dry needling, therapeutic massage, and so on.

articular cartilage, and the concentration of those large forces on that small area results in premature wear and in the pain we associate with patella-femoral syndrome. Thus, patella tracking seems to play a big role in many cases of patella-femoral syndrome. Women are built with pelvic dimensions that are typically wider than those of men. A wider pelvis results in a larger "Q angle" (Figure 1-S). The "Q" in

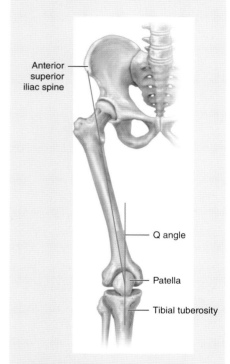

Figure 1-S. The Q (quadriceps) angle.

Q angle is for quadriceps. The force that a quadriceps muscle contraction applies to the patella is not 100% superior in its direction. The long axis of the shaft of the femur provides a good approximation of the quadriceps force vector. The largest component of this force vector is superior, but there also is a small lateral component. The greater the Q angle, the

(continued on following page)

greater the lateral force and the higher the propensity for lateral mal-tracking of the patella and consequent development of patella-femoral pain (Figure 1-T). This explains why this particular knee problem is more common in women than in men.

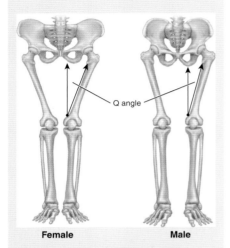

Figure 1-T. The effect of gender (pelvic width) on the Q angle.

GET LONG WHILE YOU GET STRONG

Think back to when you first learned math. If you are like most of the rest of us, learning addition was easier than learning subtraction. Why? The addition and subtraction operations are mechanically the same (but opposite). Similarly, multiplication comes easier to most of us than division. There is no logical reason why this should be either, but our brains just seem to be wired to work that way. Along the same lines, when we think about how our muscles work, we tend to think in terms of *concentric contraction*. The most classic example is the biceps curl. Imagine a sweaty, well-muscled weight lifter standing with his arms at his sides, barbells in

(continued on following page)

OR

2. **I order an MRI.** If the patient is young, this is probably a reasonable thing to do. If it comes back normal (and it is likely to come back normal in a young patient with a normal physical exam), then I give them a copy of the report (highlighting the typed words "no abnormalities found" in the conclusion at the bottom of the page) and explain that the only next step would be exploratory knee arthroscopy, which, unfortunately, has a very poor track record for improving things. I quote a statistic (i.e., half made-up and half learned from experience) that they have a 50% chance for improvement, a 30% chance of ending up about the same, and a 20% chance of being worse after exploratory surgery. If, in the back of my head, I really think they are going to do poorly and I don't want to operate on them, I'll add in the fact that medical insurance may not pay for a knee arthroscopy in a patient with no significant pathology on the MRI.

If the MRI *does* show something, then we often end up operating, but we have to explain to patients in this situation that the chances for success are diminished when the history and physical exam do not coincide with the MRI findings.

I try not to order MRIs for knee pain on patients over 65. In this age group, the incidence of abnormal findings that don't really mean anything is quite high. If, for example, you take a group of 75-year-old *asymptomatic* patients and study their knees with MRIs, the majority of them will have meniscus tears, frayed ligaments, worn articular cartilage, and a host of other findings. Because of the poor correlation between these MRI findings and meaningful pathology in older patients, our arthroscopic results are poor in this group. If confronted with a patient with "mystery knee pain" who is convinced, based on an MRI report, that he or she needs an arthroscopy, I will present the same 50%/30%/20% estimated arthroscopy outcome statistics described previously.

OR

3. **I give the patient an intra-articular cortisone injection.** The specifics of this simple, safe, and cost-effective technique are outlined in Chapter 9. The underlying pathology in some of these mystery knees is inflammatory, and the cortisone injection can work well to reduce symptoms. I will often invoke the theory of synovial impingement. Synovial impingement is a condition where a part of the synovial lining becomes pinched between the bones in the knee, and that causes that section of the lining to swell. Once it swells, it is even easier for it to become pinched a second time. The more it is pinched, the more it swells, and the more it swells, the more it tends to be pinched, producing a self-propagating cycle like the one that we've all experienced when we bite the

inside of our cheek. A single cortisone injection, I explain, can break the cycle of swelling and pinching and can solve even the most stubborn "undiagnosable" knee problem. I tell them to expect dramatic relief within 10 days and ask them to remain sedentary for that 10-day period of time (resuming strenuous activities earlier would be like biting your cheek on purpose while you are trying to let it heal).

I can't say that the guidelines I use for dealing with these mystery knees is foolproof, and you may wish to develop your own strategies, but the approach I use is safe and simple and, for the most part, cost-effective.

each hand. As he bends his right elbow and lifts the barbell up to touch his shoulder, he is performing a concentric biceps contraction. In concentric muscle contractions, the muscle shortens, bringing its origin toward its insertion. This example demonstrates a model for muscle action that anyone who has even casually studied functional anatomy will recognize. But, wait, this next part is where things get interesting. Next, the weight lifter slowly lowers the barbell back to its original position, resting at his side. Pop Quiz: What muscle did he use to return the barbell to his side? During this motion, he extends his elbow joint, and, while the biceps is the muscle that flexes the elbow joint, the *triceps* is the muscle that extends it—so, the answer is the triceps muscle. Right? WRONG! Gravity is actually pulling the weight and the lifter's arm back down to his side. If he also fired his triceps to extend his elbow during this motion, the weight would go flying down violently with the combined forces of gravity (which for a large weight can be substantial) and the triceps muscle contraction. To let the weight down slowly, the lifter needs to contract his *biceps* muscle to counteract the force of gravity trying to quickly and violently drop the weight down to its starting position. The biceps curl is actually a tug of war between gravity and the biceps muscle. The weight lifter adjusts how hard the biceps works such that the biceps wins the tug of war on the way up, and gravity wins the tug of war on the way down. The biceps is working concentrically (the muscle is shortening while it works) as the weight is raised and eccentrically (the muscle is lengthening while it works) as the weight is lowered. It has been reported that eccentric muscle progressive resistance exercises help resolve tendonitis better than concentric muscle progressive resistance exercises, so you may want to ask the physical therapists to employ eccentric exercises in the rehabilitation of a muscle with a tendon that is affected by tendonitis.

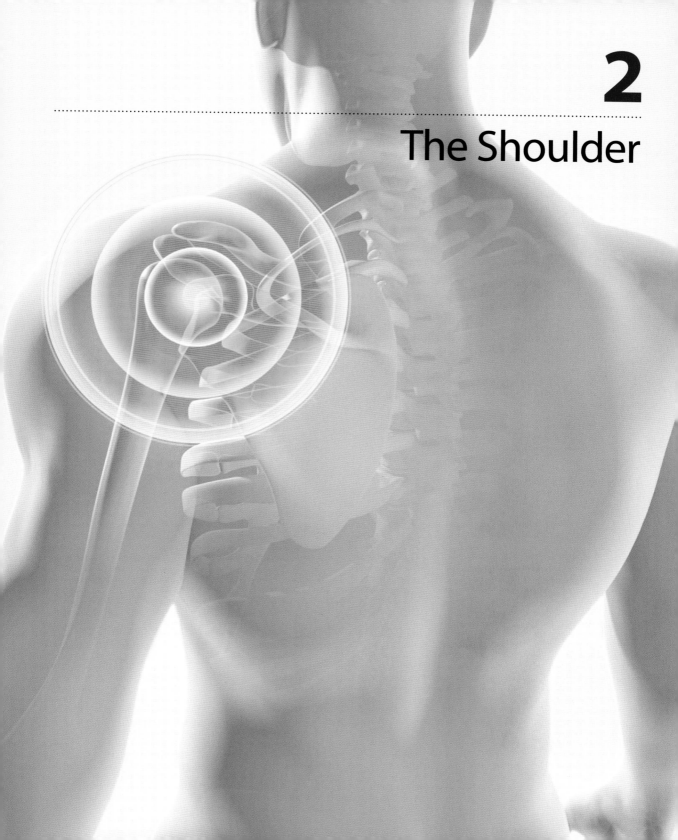

2

The Shoulder

REMEMBERING THE NAMES IS EASY ...

Remembering the names of the rotator cuff muscles is easy. Their names essentially tell us where they are located. The drawing on the left-hand side of Figure 2-2 shows the scapular spine on the posterior surface of the scapula. The muscle that originates *inferior to* the scapular spine is *infra*spinatus. The muscle that originates *superior to* the scapular spine is the *supra*spinatus (see Figure 2-6). The *subscapularis* muscle gets its name from the fact that it is on the deep surface of the scapula, underneath it and against the chest wall where it is hidden from view. You'd have to lift the scapula up off of the chest wall and look under it to see the subscapularis (Figure 2-A). The teres *minor* muscle plays a *minor* role in shoulder function or pathology. We don't need to remember where it is located.

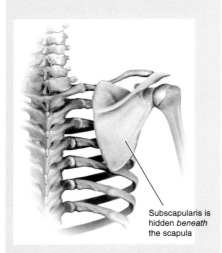

Subscapularis is hidden *beneath* the scapula

Figure 2-A. As its name implies, the subscapularis rotator cuff muscle is underneath the scapula and against the chest wall. You can't see it in a posterior view like this one because it is hidden *underneath* the scapula, hence the name: subscapularis.

As is the case with most subjects in orthopedics, the best way to start a discussion of the shoulder is to begin with the basic anatomy. This leads to some confusion right from the start because there really is no single structure that is accepted to be the "shoulder joint." In the shoulder, three bones come together to make two joints, the glenohumeral joint and the acromioclavicular (AC) joint. Technically, there is also a third articulation between the scapula and the chest wall known as the scapulothoracic joint, but pathology in the scapulothoracic joint is rare, so we will limit our discussion to the glenohumeral and AC joints. The three bones that come together to form these two joints are the clavicle, the humerus, and the scapula (Figure 2-1). Of the three bones, the

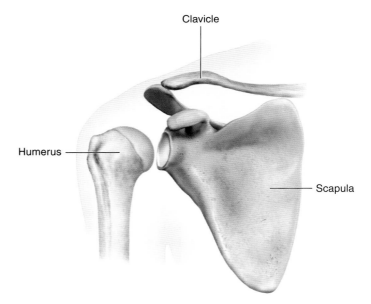

Clavicle

Humerus

Scapula

Figure 2-1. The humerus, clavicle, and scapula form the two joints of the shoulder.

scapula has the most complicated shape, so we will study it in more detail. Figure 2-2 shows the scapula viewed from three different angles: a posterior view, a lateral view, and an anterior view. Each of these views highlights a different feature of the scapula. The posterior view shows the scapular spine, a long, thin bony prominence that terminates as the acromion process. The scapular spine is a subcutaneous bony prominence that is palpable on even the heaviest patients. The lateral view shows the acromion process, the coracoid process, and the glenoid fossa. Looking at the anterior view of the shoulder gives us the best view of the coracoid process and the anterior edge of the acromion. On all of the views, we can see the thin body (blade) of the scapula. The body of the scapula is designed to provide a large surface area for the origins

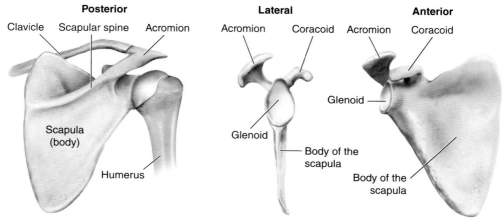

Posterior | **Lateral** | **Anterior**

Clavicle · Scapular spine · Acromion | Acromion · Coracoid | Acromion · Coracoid

Scapula (body)

Glenoid

Humerus

Glenoid

Body of the scapula

Body of the scapula

Figure 2-2. The scapula viewed from posterior (left), lateral (center), and anterior (right).

and insertions of various muscles, and, as such, it is broad and flat. The coracoid process projects anteriorly and laterally, like a hooked finger. Several tendons, including the short head of the biceps and the coracobrachialis, attach to the coracoid process.

The two joints formed by the humerus, clavicle, and scapula are stabilized by a series of firm, but flexible, ligaments (Figure 2-3).

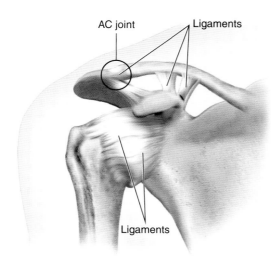

AC joint · Ligaments

Ligaments

Figure 2-3. The ligaments that stabilize the glenohumeral and acromioclavicular joints.

The ligaments that stabilize the glenohumeral joint are bands of collagen-rich connective tissue that are embedded in the substance of the joint capsule, the thick membrane that originates from the rim of the glenoid socket and inserts around the neck of the humerus.

A *LITTLE* BIOMECHANICS

In recent years, there has been a significant change in our understanding of the biomechanics of the shoulder. It wasn't that long ago that we were all taught that the function of the supraspinatus was to accomplish the first 30 degrees of shoulder abduction. In other words, if you were standing, arms at your sides, and you wanted to abduct your shoulder joints and move your arms away from your sides (think of the motion your arms make when you make a snow angel), your supraspinatus muscles would be responsible for the first 30 degrees of that motion. The reason that we thought that is how things worked is that, when patients had large supraspinatus rotator cuff tears, they lost the ability to initiate abduction. If you brought their arm out away from their side for them (past 30 degrees), they could raise it the rest of the way on their own. If they went on to have the supraspinatus tear repaired, the operation restored their ability to initiate abduction. This was observed so consistently among so many patients that it was concluded that the supraspinatus must serve to raise the arm through the first 30 degrees of abduction. We understand now that

(continued on following page)

this is not the case. To understand what's really going on here, we need to review three important facts about the structure and function of the shoulder. The first fact is that the glenoid, the socket of the ball-and-socket joint of the shoulder, isn't much of a socket at all. If you compare it to the acetabulum, the socket of the hip joint (Figure 2-B), you will see that it

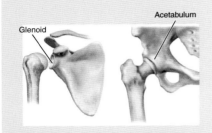

Figure 2-B. A comparison of the anatomy of the socket of the shoulder (glenoid) and the socket of the hip (acetabulum).

is much more shallow, almost like the surface of a golf tee, just a shallow dimple on which the ball rests. The second fact is that, when a patient's arm is at their side, the deltoid force vector is essentially vertical (Figure 2-C). The last fact we have to

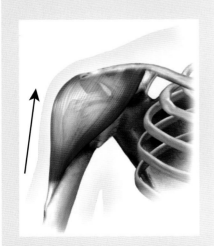

Figure 2-C. With the arm at the side, the deltoid force vector is essentially vertical.

(continued on following page)

At the point of its origin along the edge of the socket rim, the joint capsule becomes thick and dense. This tissue is known as the labrum. The AC joint has this same system of stabilizing ligaments in its capsule, but it also has an interesting, second set of ligaments that anchor the clavicle to the coracoid process. Since the coracoid process and the acromion are both part of the same bone, anchoring the clavicle to the coracoid process stabilizes the AC joint.

The next layer we encounter as we go from the deep to the superficial anatomy of the shoulder is the deepest set of shoulder muscles: the rotator cuff muscles (Figures 2-4, 2-5, 2-6, and 2-7).

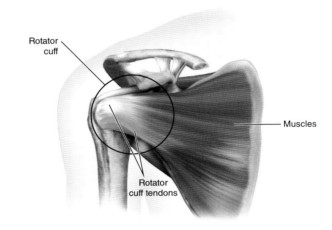

Figure 2-4. The deepest layer of muscle in the shoulder: the rotator cuff.

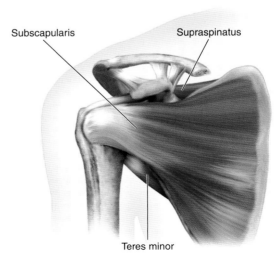

Figure 2-5. An anterior view of the shoulder showing the subscapularis and supraspinatus rotator cuff muscles.

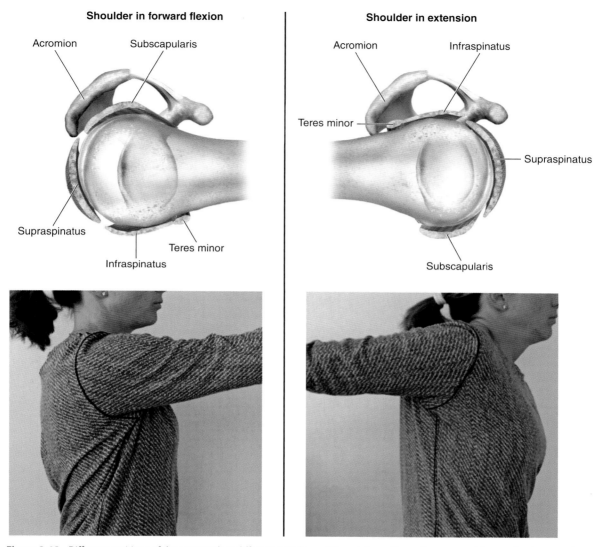

Figure 2-12. Different positions of the arm result in different members of the rotator cuff muscle group residing under the acromion.

or if a layer of calcium accumulates on the undersurface of the acromion, the subacromial space can become so narrow that the acromion bone actually strikes the bursa or rotator cuff, causing it to swell and become inflamed (Figure 2-13). The more swollen and inflamed it becomes, the more likely it is to impinge against the acromion, and the more it impinges, the more swollen and inflamed it becomes. This cycle of swelling and impinging is what creates the condition of subacromial impingement, sort of like biting the inside of your cheek creates a tender, swollen bump that makes it easier to bite it a second time, which makes it

THE GRAY HAIR AND WRINKLES OF THE SHOULDER

Rotator cuff muscle tears are interesting and unique. In most instances, when a muscle in our bodies tears, it is because

(continued on following page)

normal, healthy tissue is exposed to a sudden abnormal force. A tennis player who lunges forward to get a ball and tears his or her calf muscle would be a good example of a typical mechanism for tearing a muscle. Rotator cuff tears are different. Though it is somewhat controversial, our best data indicate that the vast majority of rotator cuff tears are *attritional* tears, and that they result from chronic abrasive wear of the rotator cuff against the underside of the acromion. Often, there is some element of trauma that is the "straw that breaks the camel's back." This can be something trivial, like lifting a sack of garbage to put it in a dumpster or throwing a ball in a recreational softball game. The trauma does cause the muscle to tear, but instead of a normal muscle tearing under an abnormal force, as was the case in the tennis player example, it is an abnormal muscle (frayed from chronic impingement) tearing when subjected to a normal force. Impingement is common, especially in older patients. As we age, it is natural for extra bone to grow and accumulate on the undersurface of the acromion. This narrows the already critically narrow subacromial space and starts the impingement process. Impingement is so common in people over 60 that it is hard to call it a pathologic condition. Like gray hair and wrinkles, it is a fact of life that most of us will have to face if we are lucky enough to live into our 60s, 70s, and beyond.

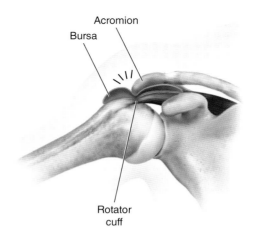

Figure 2-13. When we raise our arm forward or out to the side, the subacromial space narrows and impingement of the bursa or rotator cuff can occur.

more swollen, and so on. Subacromial space impingement is self-propagating and, as such, can become chronic. It is felt that chronic impingement of the rotator cuff against the acromion is what causes the rotator cuff to fray and eventually tear (see sidebar).

So far, we have discussed two of the occupants of the subacromial space, the subacromial bursa and the rotator cuff. The third occupant of the subacromial space is the tendon of the long head of the biceps muscle. This tendon enters the joint through a small gap between the supraspinatus and subscapularis muscles and is in a location that allows it, in certain positions of the shoulder, to impinge against the acromion (Figure 2-14). If the long-head biceps

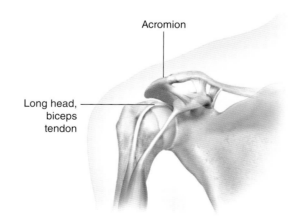

Figure 2-14. The tendon of the long head of the biceps muscle is an occupant of the subacromial space and can impinge against the underside of the acromion when the arm is raised.

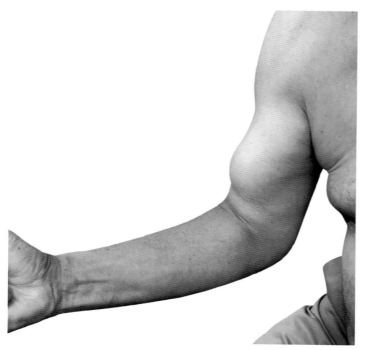

Figure 2-15. The classic "Popeye" deformity seen in patients who have sustained a rupture of the tendon of the long head of the biceps muscle from chronic subacromial impingement. Functional deficits are minimal, so surgical repair is not necessary.

LONG HEAD BICEPS TENDON RUPTURES: NO BIG DEAL

The reason ruptures of the tendon of the long head of the biceps muscle don't result in a significant strength defecit has to do with the shape of the muscle. The muscles illustrated below are both biceps (two headed) muscles. If one if the two superior heads of biceps mucle A were to rupture, all of the muscle below it would

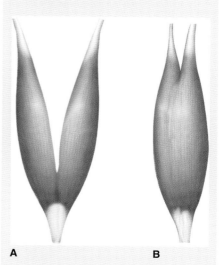

A   **B**

no longer be attached superiorly, and one would predict a profound (close to 50%) loss of strength. The human biceps looks more like biceps muscle B. If one of the two superior tendons of this mucle were to rupture, most of the muscle mass is still able to exert its force using the remaining tendon and loss of strength is minimal.

tendon becomes so damaged from impingement that it finally tears, the result is the "Popeye" deformity shown in Figure 2-15. Like most rotator cuff tears, tears of the long-head biceps tendon are typically attritional tears (see sidebar, page 51) that result from long-standing impingement against the underside of the acromion. The functional deficits that result from a long-head biceps tendon rupture are minimal (patients only lose about 5% of elbow flexion strength), so surgical repair is seldom recommended.

Subacromial space impingement is probably easiest to understand if we consider it a continuum of conditions ranging from bursitis to cuff tear arthropathy (Figure 2-16). In its early stages, it may only be the bursa that is inflamed and painful. This is the condition we refer to as subacromial bursitis or, sometimes, just "shoulder bursitis." If the condition goes on for a longer period of time, the rotator cuff (usually the supraspinatus because it spends the most time under the acromion) or the biceps tendon may become swollen and inflamed. This we know as rotator cuff or biceps tendonitis. If impingement continues, the rotator cuff or biceps tendon may rupture, resulting in a rotator cuff or biceps tendon tear. The final point on the continuum of subacromial impingement is what has been termed "cuff tear arthropathy."

CUFF TEAR ARTHROPATHY, MY DAUGHTER'S JEANS, AND THE REVERSE TOTAL SHOULDER REPLACEMENT

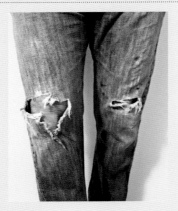

Figure 2-K. The author's daughter's favorite pair of jeans. The loss of material and frayed edges around the holes in the knees mimic the appearance of the chronic, massive rotator cuff tears seen in patients with cuff tear arthropathy.

After reading the sidebar on the biomechanics of the shoulder, you understand how important a normal rotator cuff can be to proper shoulder function. In patients with cuff tear arthropathy, there is not enough intact rotator cuff muscle to keep the humeral head pressed tightly against the glenoid socket, and the pivot point for deltoid-mediated shoulder rotation is lost. Attempts to raise the arm result in superior translation of the humeral head instead of shoulder joint rotation. Even at rest, the deltoid muscle tone translates the head of the humerus superiorly into a subluxed position above its normal location opposite the glenoid socket. Over time, the superior translation of the humeral head up against the underside of the acromion wears the underside of the acromion, causing it to have a concave geometry matching the shape of the humeral head. Figure 2-18 shows both the superior

(continued on following page)

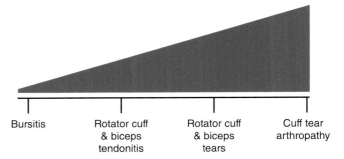

Figure 2-16. The continuum of subacromial space impingement conditions.

Figure 2-17 shows an anteroposterior (AP) x-ray of a shoulder. The occupants of the subacromial space are not visualized on a plain x-ray, so we cannot tell from this film if the patient has bursitis, a

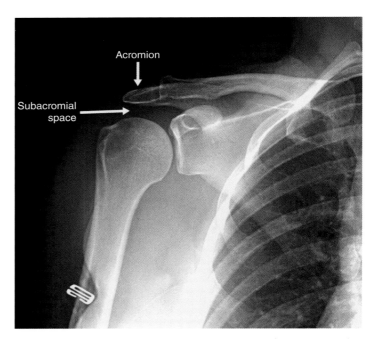

Figure 2-17. An AP x-ray of the shoulder. The occupants of the subacromial space are not visible on a plain x-ray.

rotator cuff tear, or a completely normal shoulder. Compare the x-ray in Figure 2-17 to the x-ray in Figure 2-18, which shows an x-ray of a shoulder with cuff tear arthropathy. Two major differences between the x-rays are apparent. For one, on the x-ray of the patient with cuff tear arthropathy, the humeral head is superior to its normal position opposite the glenoid socket; second, there is no

Acromion

Subacromial space

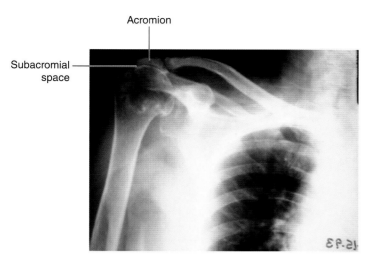

Figure 2-18. An x-ray of a shoulder with cuff tear arthropathy. The subacromial space is essentially gone. This x-ray is diagnostic of a chronic, massive rotator cuff tear.

subacromial space. The humeral head is in direct contact with the underside of the acromion. As we learned in the sidebar on shoulder biomechanics, without the rotator cuff to hold the humeral head against the glenoid socket, the superiorly directed force of the deltoid, even its resting muscle tone, causes the humeral head to translate superiorly. In cases of cuff tear arthropathy, we can make the diagnosis of a rotator cuff tear based on plain x-ray alone. It is with certainty that we can say that the cuff is torn since there is no possible way that a structure as thick as the rotator cuff can exist in the paper-thin space between the humeral head and the acromion on this x-ray. The long-head biceps tendon is likely torn as well, and what's left of the bursa, if anything, is probably severely inflamed. The appearance of the x-ray also tells us that the rotator cuff tear has been there a long time, and that it is massive. We know the process has been going on for a long time because the humeral head has ground a concavity into the underside of the acromion. Such bony changes take years to occur.

Cuff tear arthropathy is difficult to treat. The rotator cuff tear is too big to be repaired, and grafts and patches have not always worked well. An innovative solution to this problem is the reverse shoulder arthroplasty (see sidebar, page 54). This operation has revolutionized our approach to patients with this problem and helped restore function and reduce pain for a legion of patients for whom there would otherwise be no surgical solution.

▶ *Clinical Presentation: History*

Patients with impingement will typically have pain that is worse when they position their arm above their head since this is the

position of the humeral head and the abnormally shaped acromion typical in cases of cuff tear arthropathy.

Figure 2-L shows a typical rotator cuff tear on the top and one of these

A typical supraspinatus rotator cuff tear

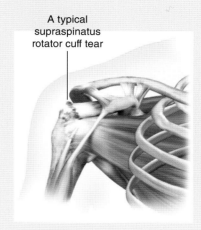

A chronic, massive rotator cuff tear

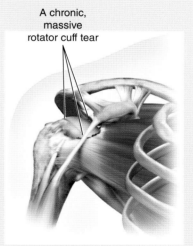

Figure 2-L. A typical rotator cuff tear (drawing on top) and chronic, massive rotator cuff tear (drawing on bottom).

massive, chronic, cuff tear arthropathy tears on the bottom. Rotator cuff tears as big and as chronic as these tears are not surgically repairable. To fix these tears, we

(continued on following page)

would have to be granted three miracles. **Miracle number one:** We would have to be able to take the leading edge of the torn rotator cuff and somehow stretch it all the way over to the lateral side of the humeral head, where it normally inserts. This would truly be a miracle. The reason it is so difficult is that this isn't just a tear; there is actually a loss of material. Furthermore, the edges of the tear are frayed and ragged and won't hold sutures well. I tell patients that this particular type of rotator cuff tear is like the holes on the knees of my teenaged daughter's favorite pair of jeans (Figure 2-K). There is a large area of missing material, and the edges of the defect are of poor quality. To accomplish a repair, we would first have to trim the edges back to healthy tissue, which would only make the already-too-big tear even bigger. We would then have to bring the

(continued on following page)

position that closes the subacromial space and pinches the bursa/biceps tendon/rotator cuff against the acromion. Of all the symptoms of impingement, pain with overhead activities is the one that is most pathognomonic, though pain when reaching behind the back is also common. It is also common for patients to complain of pain that wakes them from sleep, and the pain may radiate to the middle of the humerus, which often confuses things. Many patients with impingement don't perceive any shoulder pain at all, just pain halfway down their arm. These signs and symptoms of subacromial impingement can present identically in patients with any form of impingement: bursitis, tendonitis, or tears.

▶ Physical Exam

The best way to reproduce the shoulder pain that comes from impingement is to raise the patient's arm above their head (Figure 2-19). This is done either with the passive forward flexion test (think of the motion a football referee uses to signal a touchdown) or the passive abduction test (think of the motion you make with your arms to make a snow angel). These are both passive motion tests, meaning that the examiner raises the arm for the patient. I recommend using both tests. If one or both re-create the patient's pain, that's a sign that they have impingement syndrome.

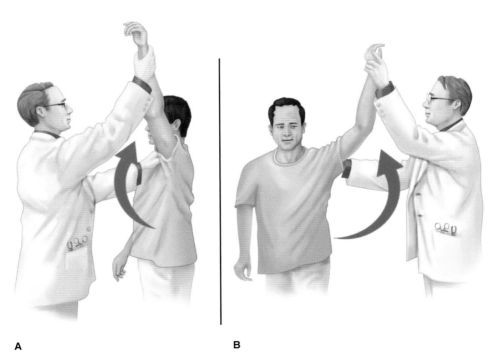

A   **B**

Figure 2-19. The forward flexion (**A**) and abduction (**B**) physical exam tests for subacromial space impingement. These are passive tests (the examiner raises the patient's arm for the patient).

Another good test is to check for tenderness to palpation over the greater tuberosity of the proximal humerus. The greater tuberosity is the structure onto which the supraspinatus and infraspinatus insert. It is directly under the subacromial bursa, and immediately lateral to the biceps tendon. This is the "neighborhood" where impingement occurs. All of the structures that become inflamed in impingement live here, in an area about the size of a quarter. The best way to check for tenderness here is to have the patient bring their arms behind their back. This brings the greater tuberosity anteriorly, out from under the acromion, where we can press on it. Test both the right and left shoulders, pressing with your thumb over the anterior shoulder (Figure 2-20). Some degree of tenderness over any bony

edges together to meet, so that we could sew them together. This would be impossible. There just isn't enough material. **Miracle number two:** The repaired rotator cuff tissue would have to heal. The sutures used to accomplish the repair will only last so long. Eventually, the only way the repair will work is if the tissue heals. Unfortunately, tissue doesn't heal well under tension, and this repair would be under massive tension. **Miracle number three:** If we are granted the first two miracles and we are able to bring the cuff over to the humerus and repair it and it heals, the result may still be poor. A proper, healthy set of rotator cuff muscles is one of the most elegant symphonies of coordinated motion found anywhere in the human body. Like firemen around a fireman's net, each member of the rotator cuff muscle group adjusts its contractile force so that the tension on the shoulder joint is balanced, and the ball stays centered in the socket regardless of the position of the shoulder and what task it is performing. It is unrealistic to expect a rotator cuff muscle that has been detached and unused for years or decades to perform in such a complicated way, and any patch-type material we use to cover the defect will not have the contractile properties of muscle, so it won't work to actively center the humeral head. So, for most of the history of the field of orthopedics, we had nothing to offer our patients with cuff tear arthropathy. Some orthopedists attempted to solve the problem by installing a conventional shoulder replacement. Unfortunately, the unopposed, superiorly directed force of the deltoid in a rotator cuff–deficient *artificial* shoulder is no different from that in a cuff-deficient native shoulder, and the artificial ball also subluxes superiorly out of the artificial socket to rest against the underside of the acromion (Figure 2-M). In an attempt to prevent superior humeral head subluxation, designs of an artificial

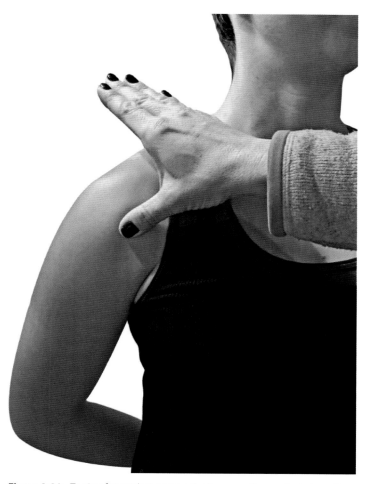

Figure 2-20. Testing for tenderness to palpation over the greater tuberosity of the proximal humerus.

(continued on following page)

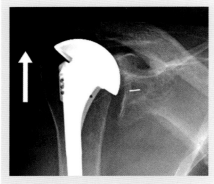

Figure 2-M. A conventional artificial shoulder in a rotator cuff–deficient patient. Note that the artificial humeral head has subluxed out of the socket superiorly due to the unopposed superiorly directed force of the deltoid muscle (*Reproduced with permission from Armand Hatzidakis, MD*).

glenoid with a larger superior lip were considered (Figure 2-N), but when the humeral head would ride up against the superior lip of the device, a tilting force developed that tended to loosen the bond that held the artificial glenoid to

(continued on following page)

prominence is normal, but, if the bursa, biceps, or rotator cuff is inflamed, the affected shoulder will be significantly more tender than the asymptomatic shoulder.

The strength of each of the three rotator cuff muscles (remember, we're going to forget about teres minor) should be assessed. The easiest way to do this is to apply three different tests, one for subscapularis, one for infraspinatus, and one for supraspinatus. Have the patient start with their arms at their sides, elbows bent 90 degrees (Figure 2-21). Ask them to keep their elbows at their sides and rotate their forearms out as far as they can. Now have them perform the same motion, but this time have them rotate out while pushing their wrists against the palms of your hands while you push in to resist them. This is an active motion test (the patient performs the motion, not the examiner). This particular test, active external rotation against resistance, tests the member of the rotator cuff muscle group that is responsible for external rotation of the shoulder, the infraspinatus. To test the subscapularis, simply apply the same test in the opposite direction, having the patient press in toward the midline against your resistance. This is a good, but not great, test of subscapularis function. Because the pectoral muscles also participate in resisted internal rotation in this position, tests like the belly press test and the lift-off test (Figure 2-22) yield a more precise assessment of subscapularis strength, but internal rotation against resistance with the elbow at the side will suffice for most clinical situations.

The tests used to measure the strength of infraspinatus and subscapularis make sense. To test a muscle that is an external

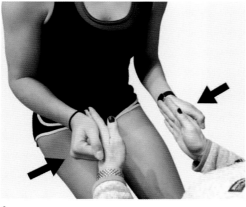

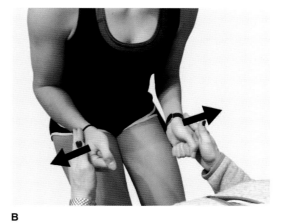

A   **B**

Figure 2-21. Using internal (**A**) and external (**B**) rotation against resistance to test the strength of subscapularis and infraspinatus. Subscapularis is tested by having the patient push in, toward the midline, against the resistance of the examiner, who is pushing out, away from the midline. This is illustrated in the photograph in (**A**). Infraspinatus is tested by having the patient push out, away from the midline, against the resistance of the examiner, who is pushing in, toward the midline (**B**).

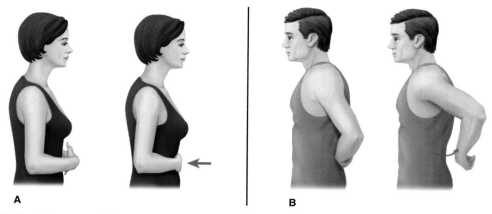

Figure 2-22. The belly press test (**A**) tests the subscapularis by having the patient press the palm of their hand against their abdomen. Patients with subscapularis pathology will have difficulty pressing firmly due to subscapularis weakness. Patients with a weak or injured subscapularis cannot press their palm firmly onto their abdomen. The lift-off test (**B**) tests the subscapularis by determining if the patient can lift their hand off their back. This is difficult without an intact subscapularis rotator cuff muscle.

rotator, we have the patient externally rotate against resistance. To test a muscle that is an internal rotator, we have the patient internally rotate against resistance. The test for supraspinatus isn't as obvious, but it has a great name: "the empty can test," which helps make it easy to remember. Before it was introduced, everyone agreed on the internal and external rotation tests for subscapularis and infraspinatus, but there was no consensus opinion regarding which test to use for supraspinatus. That was a big problem because the supraspinatus is the muscle most often affected by impingement and, as such, the most important one to test.

Jobe and Moynes are credited with using electromyographic (EMG) data to compare different proposed supraspinatus strength tests. Their research indicated that the empty can test was the physical exam maneuver that best assessed supraspinatus function. To perform the test, have the patient stand with their arms stretched out in front of them, thumbs down, like each hand is pouring the contents of a can out onto the floor in front of them. The elbows should be locked out straight into full extension, and the arms should be angled slightly down toward the ground (Figure 2-23).

Based on the results of the physical exam, we can (a) determine if our patient with shoulder pain has impingement and (b) determine the degree of impingement they have (see sidebar, page 62).

▶ *Imaging*

The x-ray view that is most helpful in evaluating a patient with impingement is the "Y view" or, its close cousin, the "outlet view." The Y view is taken with the beam of the x-ray approximately parallel to the scapular spine and the film against the anterior

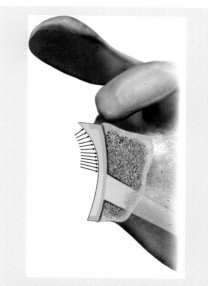

Figure 2-N. An artificial glenoid design with a large superior lip to try to contain the humerus in a rotator cuff–deficient shoulder. These designs were abandoned due to the high leverage forces they apply to the interface between the artificial glenoid and the scapula, resulting in premature failure of the bond between the part and the bone.

(continued on following page)

the scapula (think of pressing down on the rim of your dinner plate. The plate flips up as a result of the tilting force your fingers apply to the plate). For decades, we struggled with addressing the needs of patients with cuff tear arthropathy and were not able to offer any meaningful solutions until the recent introduction of a new and novel type of shoulder joint replacement called the reverse total shoulder. The operation gets its name from the fact that the ball is placed on the scapula and the socket is placed on the humerus (Figures 2-O and 2-P).

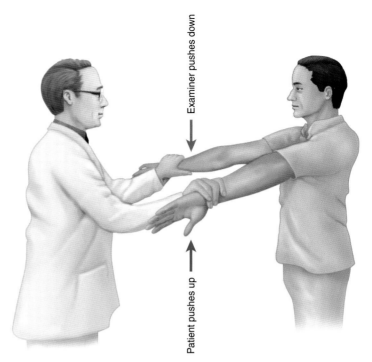

Examiner pushes down

Patient pushes up

Figure 2-23. The "empty can test" used to assess supraspinatus strength. The patient pushes up against the resistance of the examiner, who is pushing down.

shoulder (Figure 2-24). Figure 2-25 shows how the scapula looks like the letter Y when viewed from this direction, and Figure 2-26 shows a large subacromial spur on the underside of the acromion, as seen on a Y-view x-ray. It is not uncommon to see large bone

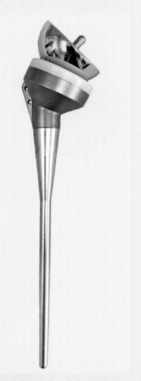

Figure 2-O. The reverse total shoulder replacement. In this design, the ball is attached to the scapula, the humeral head is removed, and the socket is attached to the top of the humerus (*Reproduced with permission from Armand Hatzidakis, MD*).

(continued on following page)

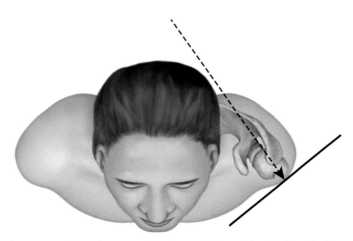

Figure 2-24. The technique used to obtain a Y view of the shoulder. The Y view allows us to peer underneath the acromion into the subacromial space.

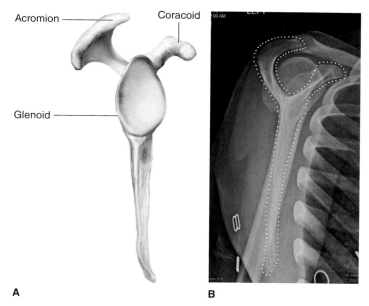

A

B

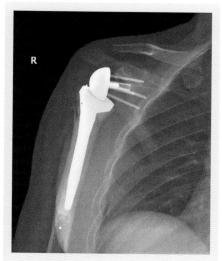

Figure 2-P. An x-ray showing a reverse shoulder replacement in a patient with a rotator cuff–deficient shoulder (*Reproduced with permission from Armand Hatzidakis, MD*).

Figure 2-25. The Y view is essentially a lateral view of the scapula. From this angle, the body, scapular spine, and coracoid process form a *Y*. The glenoid socket is centered where the three limbs of the Y intersect.

As the deltoid contracts, the humerus cannot translate superiorly because the ball bonded to the scapula is there to stop it. The socket-shaped humeral component glides along the surface of the ball, and the shoulder rotates. The procedure is relatively new, and there are concerns about forces at the ball/scapula interface causing premature loosening, but so far the device appears to be performing well without the problems that the lipped glenoid and other designs had experienced.

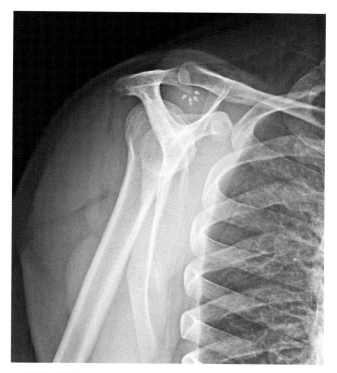

Figure 2-26. A Y view in a patient showing a large spur on the undersurface of the acromion (arrows).

WHERE ARE YOU ON THE CONTINUUM?

Figure 2-16 shows a continuum of conditions, all of which are considered to be in the "family" of subacromial impingement. The least-severe impingement conditions are on the left, the most severe on the right. Using the simple physical exam tests discussed in this chapter, we can attempt to determine where our patients are along this continuum. For instance, suppose you recreate the patient's pain when you raise

(continued on following page)

spurs like this one in older patients (see sidebar, page 51). In most cases, x-rays aren't necessary for the average patient in an outpatient setting who has impingement. They help identify arthritis (a different source of shoulder pain, to be discussed further in the chapter), and they show the bony changes associated with cuff tear arthropathy, but these conditions can often be diagnosed based on history and physical exam.

Magnetic resonance imaging (MRI) is a sensitive and specific test for evaluating the shoulder, but it is an expensive test, and as discussed in the treatment section that follows, it is often unnecessary. Figure 2-27 shows a drawing and coronal MRI images of the shoulder demonstrating the supraspinatus passing through the subacromial space. The lower MRI image shows a supraspinatus rotator cuff tear (small arrow). Figure 2-28 shows a narrow subacromial space and supraspinatus impingement without a tear.

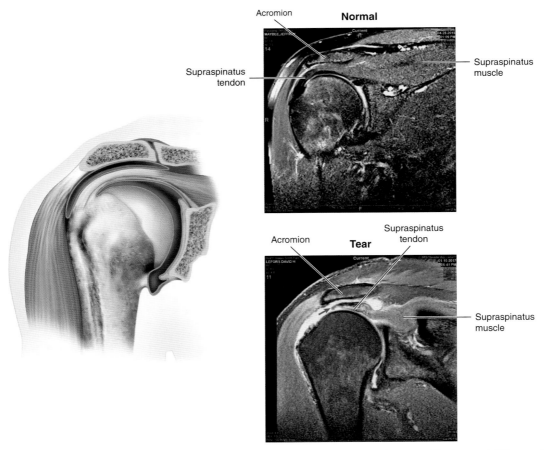

Figure 2-27. A drawing (left) and two coronal MRI images. The top MRI image shows normal anatomy. The bottom MRI image shows a supraspinatus rotator cuff tear (small arrows) (*MRI images reproduced with permission from Armand Hatzidakis, MD*).

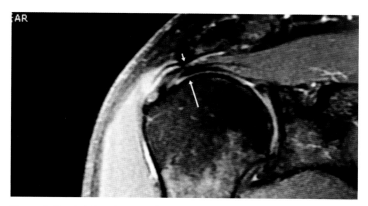

Figure 2-28. A tight subacromial space resulting in impingement of the supraspinatus (arrows).

▶ *Medical Treatment*

Fortunately, most cases of subacromial space impingement can be treated nonoperatively. Nonsteroidal anti-inflammatory drugs (NSAIDs) can help. They decrease inflammation in the bursa, rotator cuff, and biceps. This reduces swelling in these structures and can allow them to glide beneath the acromion without impinging against it. Physical therapy can help as well, but be careful. If we don't adequately communicate the diagnosis to the therapist, they may start range-of-motion exercises that can worsen impingement. The commonly used physical therapy home exercise where the patient uses their fingers to "walk their hand up the wall," for instance, subjects the occupants of the subacromial space to repeated impingement events as the arm is placed repeatedly in the overhead position.

Attempts should be made to maintain and, later, increase range of motion through the pain-free part of the patient's arc of shoulder motion. Specific strength exercises are helpful for impingement. Shoulders with injured, inflamed, malfunctioning rotator cuff muscles tend to have a humeral head that resides superior to its normal position directly lateral to the glenoid socket (see sidebar A *Little* Biomechanics). This further narrows the subacromial space and makes impingement matters worse. A physical therapy program aimed at strengthening the subscapularis and infraspinatus muscles (both of which have a downward force vector, as shown in Figure 2-29) can help bring the humeral head back down where it belongs and increase the subacromial space. These muscles can be strengthened with internal and external rotation exercises using weights, weighted cables, or simply isometric contraction (rotating the arm in or out against a wall or a door jam). It is important for the arm to be down by the patient's side while these exercises are performed to avoid further impingement. So, when writing a physical therapy prescription for this condition, be sure to list subacromial impingement as the diagnosis. Ask the

their arm above them in forward flexion (Figure 2-19A) or abduction (Figure 2-19B). Also, assume that they are tender over the greater tuberosity of the proximal humerus with their arm behind their back (Figure 2-20). This certainly is starting to look like a patient with subacromial space impingement. Now, suppose they have no pain or weakness on any of the rotator cuff strength tests. Where are they on the impingement continuum? It would be reasonable to deduce that they have bursitis. In this condition, the bursa is swollen, irritated and inflamed, and it becomes pinched between the humeral head and the underside of the acromion when the arm is raised. There is no pain when the arm is at the side. Because the rotator cuff is not affected and we perform our strength tests in positions of the arm where the subacromial space is wide open, the patient has normal rotator cuff strength as assessed by the internal rotation against resistance (subscapularis) test, the external rotation against resistance (infraspinatus) test, and the empty can (supraspinatus) test. Remember, these rotator cuff strength tests are administered *with the patient's arms low and the subacromial space open*. With the subacromial space wide open, none of its occupants are pinched against the underside of the acromion. Not only do they not have any weakness when we administer these strength tests, but also they have no pain (remember, in bursitis, only the bursa is inflamed; the muscles are normal). If a different patient has identical physical exam findings when we raise their arm (it hurts), is also tender over the greater tuberosity, *but has both pain and weakness on the empty can test,* then we know that this second patient has more than just bursitis. The supraspinatus is involved. We don't know if it is torn or just inflamed, but the positive empty can test tells us that the supraspinatus is involved. It is injured, and it hurts to

(continued on following page)

contract it, even if the arm is at the side, where the acromion isn't impinging against anything. If we want to go one step further toward solving this puzzle, we can inject the subacromial space with lidocaine (or a cortisone injection *that contains lidocaine*). If we retest the patient after the injection and their pain goes away and their weakness resolves, we would deduce that they have supraspinatus rotator cuff *tendonitis*. In the strength test before the lidocaine injection, they were weak because the muscle hurt. It wasn't torn; it just hurt too much to contract. With the lidocaine in the subacromial space to deaden the discomfort, the muscle is strong when tested after the injection. Now, consider a third scenario. Imagine a patient identical to the patient in the second example, but in this patient, the lidocaine injection has a different effect. When we test this third patient after administering the injection of lidocaine into the subacromial space, the pain goes away, but the weakness on the empty can test persists. This patient may have a supraspinatus tear. The lidocaine can take away the pain, but it cannot repair the tear, so the weakness persists when the patient is retested after the injection.

So, with three simple strength tests and a few milliliters of lidocaine (see the technique on subacromial space injections in Chapter 9), we not only can diagnose impingement but also can try to see where on the continuum of impingement our patients are. This is why we test internal and external rotation *with the patient's arms at their sides,* and we perform the empty can test with the *outstretched arms pointing slightly down toward the floor.* If we test rotator cuff strength with the arms raised, the impingement of an inflamed bursa that occurs in this position could cause enough pain to produce weakness, invalidating our strength tests. These tests aren't perfect, but they can help us try to understand how severe a patient's impingement is and what structures are involved.

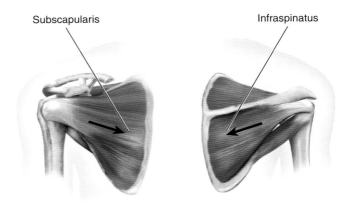

Figure 2-29. The downward force that the subscapularis and infraspinatus rotator cuff muscles exert on the humeral head may help keep the head from migrating superiorly.

therapist to strengthen the infraspinatus and subscapularis muscles and to work on scapular retraction (proper posture can open the subacromial space) and have them limit range-of-motion exercises to areas in the arc of motion that are pain free.

If a month of NSAIDs and physical therapy exercises fail to produce an effect, a good next step is a cortisone injection into the subacromial space (see Chapter 9 to learn this technique). By decreasing inflammation in the subacromial space and reducing swelling, the injection can reduce the dimensions of the inflamed bursa, rotator cuff, or biceps tendon and relieve impingement. Within a few days to a week after the injection, one of four results will occur:

1. **The patient gets better and stays better.** This is the best-case scenario. Corticosteroids are known to cause atrophy of adipose tissue, and if this atrophy results in increasing the volume of the subacromial space, then it could result in a permanent resolution of impingement symptoms.

2. **The patient gets better for a long time (longer than 4 months) and then the symptoms return.** For these patients, a repeat cortisone injection is an option. You may see patients in your practice who have infrequent bouts of recurrent impingement (from hanging the Christmas lights or doing a project where they have to reach overhead repeatedly). If they respond well to injections, they can be managed safely with them. There is a consensus opinion that cortisone should not be repeated too frequently due to concerns of steroid toxicity to tendons and other connective tissue structures. A safe bet is not to inject more than once every 4 months.

3. **They get nothing out of the injection, not even a day of relief.** I recommend an MRI for these patients. They may have a shoulder condition that isn't impingement, and the MRI can help us identify that.

4. **They get better, but only for a short time (less than 4 months).**
   These patients are good candidates for surgery. The fact that
   they got better confirms that they have impingement, and if
   they are symptomatic before 4 months have passed, then it
   is too soon to administer another injection. These patients
   can benefit from a subacromial decompression operation
   to open up the subacromial space. Without surgery, if they
   continue to impinge, they may proceed down the continuum
   of impingement (see Figure 2-16), potentially with cuff tears
   and arthropathy, and the further they go, the more involved
   treatment becomes.

▶ Surgical Treatment

The surgical treatment for subacromial space impingement is a
subacromial decompression. This is a simple outpatient procedure
in which an arthroscope and arthroscopic tools are introduced into
the shoulder, and the underside of the acromion bone is removed
to increase the dimensions of the subacromial space. It is not necessary to know going into this surgery if the cuff is torn. That can
be determined (and determined more accurately with arthroscopic
inspection than with an MRI) during surgery. If there is no tear,
then the subacromial decompression will suffice. If there is a tear, it
can be repaired during the same operation. Figure 2-30 is a drawing

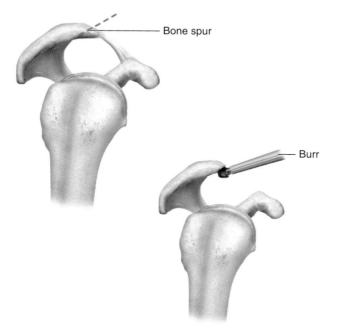

Bone spur

Burr

Figure 2-30. A drawing showing the use of an arthroscopic burr to remove
the underside of the acromion during an arthroscopic subacromial decompression procedure.

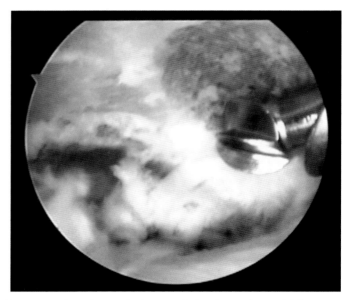

Figure 2-31. An arthroscopic photograph showing a subacromial decompression in progress.

that shows an arthroscopic burr being used to remove the underside of the acromion. Figure 2-31 is an arthroscopic photograph of the same procedure. Figure 2-32 shows how an intact rotator cuff (A) and torn rotator cuff (B) appear arthroscopically. In Figure 2-32, the arthroscope is in the glenohumeral joint, and we are looking up at the undersurface of the supraspinatus where it attaches to the humerus. The arrows in B show the tear. Figure 2-33 shows a supraspinatus rotator cuff tear (most common) and the suture repair used to fix

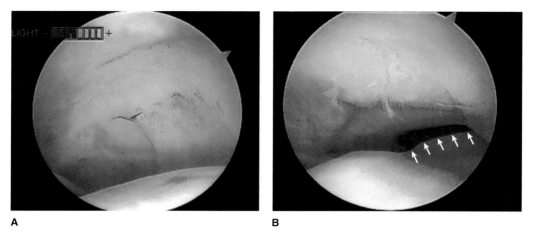

A   **B**

Figure 2-32. Arthroscopic photographs showing an intact rotator cuff (left) and a torn rotator cuff (right).

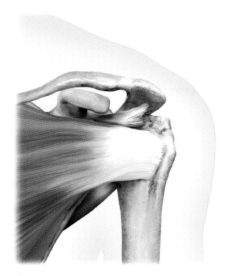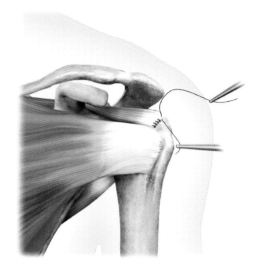

Figure 2-33. Repairing a supraspinatus rotator cuff tear.

it. The rotator cuff repair can be done through an open incision or arthroscopically. Again, our best results are with patients who responded well, but temporarily, to a subacromial injection. Surgical results are mixed, at best, in patients whose tears are so big that they aren't easily repaired and patients who are elderly and don't heal their repairs as well as younger patients.

GLENOHUMERAL JOINT INSTABILITY (SHOULDER DISLOCATION)

Glenohumeral joint dislocations are rarely seen in an outpatient setting, and they are discussed here for the sake of completeness. Feel free to skip ahead or read on if you are curious.

Like any joint, the two joints of the shoulder (the glenohumeral and AC joints) can dislocate. When the AC joint dislocates, we call it an AC joint separation, and AC joint separations are discussed separately in the following material. Figure 2-34 shows a glenohumeral joint dislocation. Look at it for a minute. Is this an anterior or a posterior dislocation? Can you tell? The truth is, you cannot tell from a single AP x-ray. The ball is definitely out of the socket, and it is inferior to it, but it could be anteriorly or posteriorly dislocated. You just can't tell. If you play the odds, the safe guess is anterior.

Over 90% of shoulder dislocations are anterior dislocations (Figure 2-35). To know for sure, we need to shoot a Y-view x-ray (see Figure 2-24 to review how this x-ray is taken). Figure 2-36 is a Y-view x-ray of the dislocation seen in Figure 2-34. With the humerus dislocated, we have an unobstructed view of the scapula, and we can see that it really does look like a *Y* viewed from

WHO WINS THE TUG-OF-WAR?

Posterior dislocations of the glenohumeral joint are rare, but when they do occur, they are commonly the result of one of two conditions: a grand mal seizure or an electrocution injury. In both of these conditions, the muscles around the glenohumeral joint all undergo a simultaneous, maximal contraction. The strongest muscles are in the back, so if all of the shoulder muscles are contracting as hard as they can, all at once, the stronger posterior muscles win the "tug-of-war," and the humeral head comes out posteriorly. The Y-view x-ray is a great x-ray for evaluating patients in whom you suspect a shoulder dislocation. It is easy

(continued on following page)

to do, and it doesn't require the patient to put the arm in a position that might be uncomfortable for them. It can even be taken with the patient's arm in a sling if necessary. A good rule of thumb is that the center of the Y should be somewhere within the outline of the humeral head on a Y-view x-ray. If it is not, then the patient has a glenohumeral joint dislocation. On a Y-view x-ray, anterior dislocations (Figure 2-36) and posterior dislocations (Figure 2-Q) are fairly easy to distinguish.

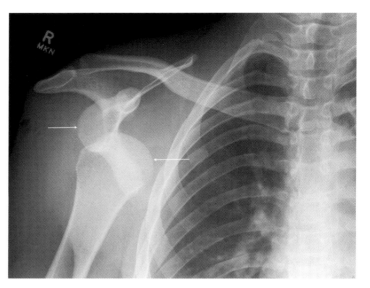

Figure 2-34. An AP x-ray showing a glenohumeral joint dislocation (arrows) (*Reproduced with permission from Armand Hatzidakis, MD*).

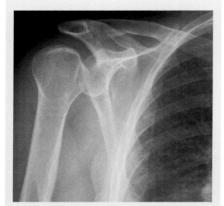

Figure 2-Q. A Y-view x-ray showing a posterior shoulder glenohumeral joint dislocation (*Reproduced with permission from Armand Hatzidakis, MD*).

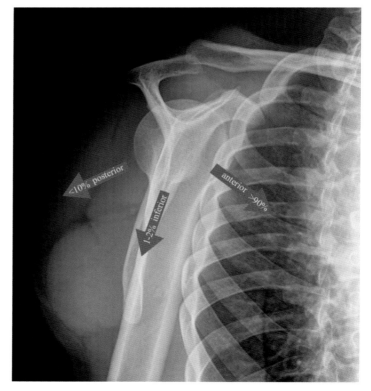

Figure 2-35. A Y-view x-ray showing the different possible directions for glenohumeral dislocations and their approximate frequencies.

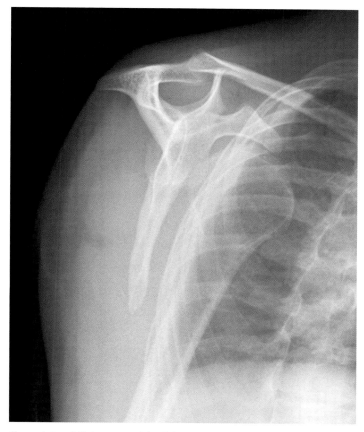

Figure 2-36. A Y-view x-ray of the dislocation shown in Figure 2-34 confirming that the dislocation is anterior (the most common direction for glenohumeral joint dislocations).

this direction. In the example in Figure 2-36, the humeral head is right under the coracoid process of the scapula (see Figure 2-2 for a quick review of this anatomy), and the coracoid is an anterior structure, so we know that this shoulder dislocation is an anterior dislocation.

There is a reason anterior dislocations are so common. If we look at the shoulder from above (Figure 2-37), we see that the joint surface of the glenoid socket is at an angle compared to the front of the body. In other words, an arrow passing through the joint is not perpendicular to the coronal plane (dotted line), but at 45 degrees to it. With the glenoid socket angled this way, there is plenty of socket bone medial and posterior to the humeral head, but no bone at all anterior to it. With no bone in front to stop it, the humeral head tends to dislocate anteriorly more than it does in any other direction.

True, complete superior dislocations (not the superior sub-luxations like the one in Figure 2-18 that we see with rotator cuff

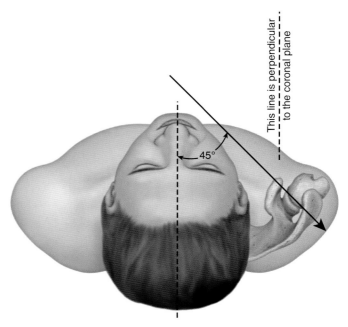

Figure 2-37. An arrow passing through the glenohumeral joint parallel to the articular surface of the glenoid socket is not perpendicular to the coronal plane, but at a 45-degree angle.

deficiency, but complete superior dislocations) are impossible because the acromion is there to block the humeral head from dislocating out the top. Inferior dislocations are extremely rare, but when they occur, can have devastating consequences. The axillary artery, vein, and brachial plexus all reside in the axilla and can be injured when the humeral head is dislocated inferiorly. Posterior dislocations are the second most common form of glenohumeral joint dislocation but are still much less common than anterior dislocations (see sidebar, page 67).

The treatment of an acute glenohumeral joint dislocation is immediate relocation. Whether this is practical in an office setting depends on a number of factors, including the comfort level of the provider and the pain tolerance of the patient. In most instances, it may be safer and more efficient to refer the patient to the emergency department, where tools such as intravenous sedation, proper airway management, and x-ray are available.

GLENOHUMERAL JOINT ARTHRITIS

The surface of the humeral head and the surface of the glenoid socket are both coated with a thin layer of slick, numb articular cartilage (see The Miracle of Gristle sidebar in Chapter 1, page 18). This layer of tissue provides ideal bearing surfaces for smooth, pain-free motion of the shoulder joint. Unfortunately, like the cartilage surfaces in all joints, it has no ability to heal or regenerate, so, over time, as we accumulate joint wear and tear, it becomes thinner and thinner. If we wear all the way through the articular cartilage down to the bone beneath it, then we expose a raw surface of bone, and that raw surface of rough, sensitive bone becomes the bearing surface of the shoulder joint. Because it is rough and sensitive, it is a poor bearing surface, and shoulders that have lost their articular cartilage surfaces are stiff and uncomfortable. As discussed in Chapter 1, the process of losing cartilage down to bone is called arthritis and can be the result of wear and tear, a rheumatic disease, infection, or trauma. Patients at risk are the elderly, patients who have had significant shoulder trauma, and patients with a long history of overuse (in sports, work, or both). Regardless of the etiology, the result is the same: a stiff, painful shoulder. Figure 2-38 shows the articular surface of a humeral

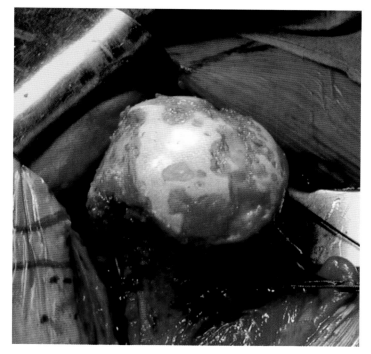

Figure 2-38. A photograph showing down to bone arthritis on the surface of the humeral head. The exposed bone is richly innervated, rough, and abrasive, resulting in a shoulder joint that is stiff and painful.

head with advanced arthritis. The articular surface cartilage has worn away, exposing large areas of rough, sensitive bone.

▶ Physical Exam

Patients with glenohumeral joint arthritis complain of pain and stiffness, but these complaints are not very specific. Our best tools

WHO STUCK MY SHEETS TOGETHER?!?

In the main text, we discuss the importance of checking range of motion with the patient's arms at their sides as a test for glenohumeral arthritis. If the passive external rotation range of motion of the affected side is poor and testing produces pain, the most likely diagnosis is glenohumeral joint arthritis. But, there is another condition that can produce this clinical finding: adhesive capsulitis. The layers of muscles that envelop the shoulder are layered on top of each other like the sheets on your bed, and to work properly, they need to glide independently back and forth like the sheets on your bed. In adhesive capsulitis, adjacent layers become stuck together by abnormal connections called adhesions. The adhesions limit the excursion of these tissue layers, and the result is stiffness *in every direction*. Because it hurts to pull against these adhesions, patients with adhesive capsulitis will have pain at the ends of their range-of-motion limits. If we are testing abduction or forward flexion by raising their arm up over their head, the pain this physical exam maneuver produces can mislead us into thinking they have impingement. When we test internal and external rotation range of motion with their arms at their sides, we encounter external rotation stiffness and think: "Aha! Glenohumeral joint arthritis!" But, the x-rays are normal, with no trace of joint space narrowing. These findings are typical of a patient with adhesive capsulitis. Fortunately, most patients with adhesive capsulitis get better with a physical therapy program concentrating on progressive stretching, but it can take months. In the few cases that don't respond, a manipulation under anesthesia to break apart the adhesions can help.

for making this diagnosis are the physical exam and a properly taken set of x-rays. On physical examination, patients with glenohumeral arthritis may have pain and stiffness that limit them when they attempt to raise their arm above their head. If we stopped the exam at this point, we might think that the diagnosis is subacromial space impingement. The key to diagnosing glenohumeral arthritis is then to check the patient's *passive* internal and external rotation range of motion with their elbows at their sides. Patients with impingement are comfortable in this position because, with the elbows at the side, the subacromial space is wide open, and impingement does not typically occur here. You will be able to rotate the shoulder of a patient with an impingement from full internal rotation (with their palm on their stomach) to full external rotation (usually about 90 degrees from the starting position; Figure 2-39) without encountering any pain or stiffness.

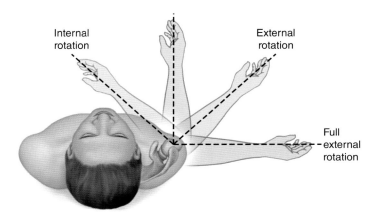

Figure 2-39. Internal and external rotation of the shoulder joint viewed from above.

A patient with glenohumeral joint arthritis will have a very different exam. Usually internal rotation is preserved, but they almost always have profound stiffness and significant discomfort with external rotation past about 30 degrees. To test for this, have them sit on the exam table facing you with their elbows bent 90 degrees, arms at their sides. Slowly rotate their forearms, one at a time, through an internal/external rotation range of motion. This test is similar to the internal/external rotation test we learned for assessing subscapularis and infraspinatus strength, but that test involved *active* motion (the patient used *their* muscles to rotate the shoulder). In this test, we are checking *passive* motion (the patient's muscles are relaxed and we, the examiner, are rotating the shoulder for them). If they have glenohumeral joint arthritis of any clinical significance, their affected shoulder won't externally rotate very well due to stiffness and pain. If you put your other hand on their shoulder as you examine them, you may feel crepitus as the bones grate against each other. The other common condition that can result in this exam finding of stiffness with passive internal and external rotation testing is adhesive capsulitis (see sidebar, page 72). This condition is also known as the "frozen shoulder" and is an important condition to know and understand. Take the time to read the sidebar on page 72; I think you'll find it useful.

▶ *Imaging*

It can be difficult to differentiate adhesive capsulitis from glenohumeral arthritis on physical exam alone. Looking for joint space narrowing on an x-ray of the shoulder can help. Arthritic shoulders will have joint space narrowing on x-ray; shoulders with adhesive capsulitis will not. The best views to use to look for narrowing of the glenohumeral joint space are the axillary and AP views. Figure 2-40 shows how the patient is positioned for an axillary view

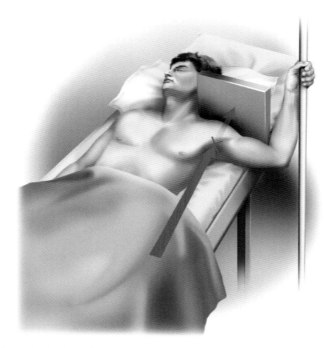

Figure 2-40. The technique used to take an axillary view x-ray of the left shoulder. The red arrow represents the x-ray beam.

x-ray. Figure 2-41 is an example of a normal axillary view, showing a well-preserved joint space between the humeral head and the

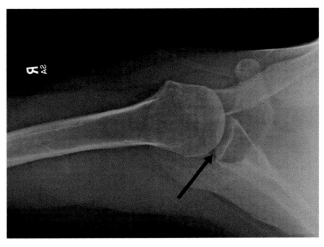

Figure 2-41. An axillary view x-ray of the right shoulder showing a normal (no arthritis) joint space between the humeral head and the glenoid socket (arrow).

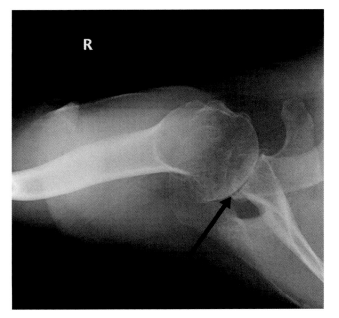

Figure 2-42. An axillary view x-ray showing bone-on-bone arthritis of the glenohumeral joint (arrow).

glenoid socket (arrow). The arrow in Figure 2-42 shows how bone-on-bone arthritis appears on this view. The AP view can also be used to diagnose glenohumeral joint arthritis. Figure 2-43 shows bone-on-bone arthritis (left) and a normal joint space (right).

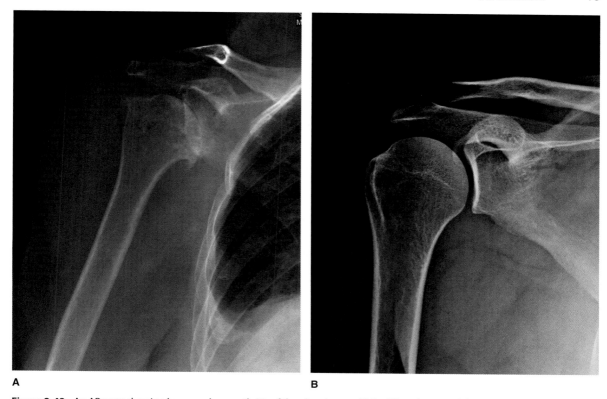

Figure 2-43. An AP x-ray showing bone-on-bone arthritis of the glenohumeral joint (**A**) and a normal shoulder (**B**).

To optimize our ability to evaluate the glenohumeral joint space on an AP x-ray, care must be taken to position the patient properly. Most AP views of the shoulder aren't AP views at all. They are taken the way you would take an AP of the chest, with the x-ray beam perpendicular to the coronal plane. This results in an oblique view of the glenohumeral joint (Figure 2-44). Figure 2-45 shows a better technique for obtaining a true AP of the glenohumeral joint. Radiology technicians refer to this "proper AP" x-ray view of the glenohumeral joint as a *Grashey* view, and most of them can provide you with this view if you order it by that name.

▶ Medical Treatment

NSAIDs and a physical therapy program intended to stretch the glenohumeral joint capsule and increase flexibility are effective in many patients. Since the shoulder is a non–weight-bearing joint, patients tend to tolerate shoulder arthritis better than arthritis of the hips or knees, and nonoperative management succeeds more often. A cortisone injection into the glenohumeral joint can also be effective (see Chapter 9 for details on how to administer this injection).

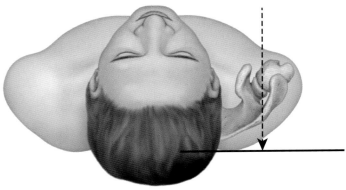

A

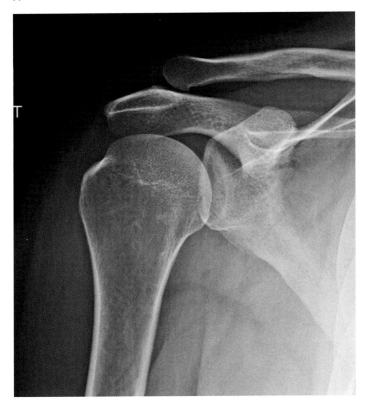

B

Figure 2-44. An improper technique for taking an AP x-ray of the shoulder (**A**). The x-ray beam is perpendicular to the coronal plane, resulting in an oblique view of the glenohumeral joint (**B**).

▶ *Surgical Treatment*

The symptoms of pain and stiffness that are typical of glenohumeral joint arthritis result from the fact that the humeral head and glenoid socket have both lost their numb, slick layers of articular

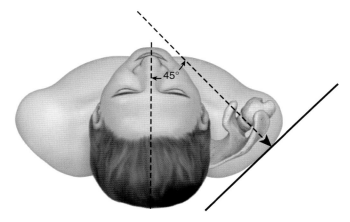

A

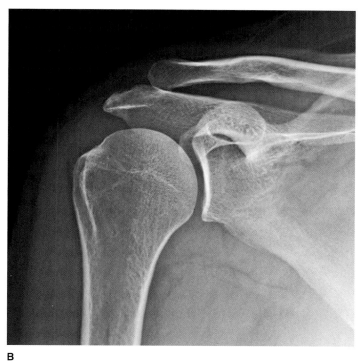

B

Figure 2-45. The technique for taking a proper AP view of the shoulder, also known as a Grashey view (**A**). The x-ray beam is oriented 45 degrees to the coronal plane, giving us a better image of the space between the humeral head and glenoid socket (**B**).

cartilage. The surgical solution to this problem is to resurface them both with materials that are slick, numb, and durable. Currently, this is accomplished by performing a shoulder joint replacement (Figure 2-46).

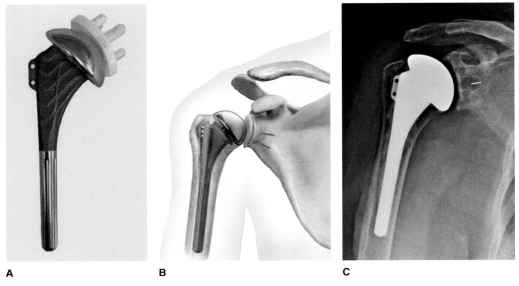

A   **B**   **C**

Figure 2-46. A typical shoulder replacement. The device is shown in **A** and **B** and its appearance on x-ray is shown in **C**. Note that the plastic piece that is used to resurface the glenoid does not show up on x-ray. It does create a lucent "gap" between the glenoid surface and the metal humeral head. (*Sample device and x-ray image reproduced with permission from Armand Hatzidakis, MD*).

In this operation, we bond a polyethylene plastic socket surface to the glenoid fossa and bond a polished metal ball to the top of the humerus. The native, arthritic humeral head is removed, and the metal dome that replaces it is anchored to the shaft of the humerus with a stem that is inserted into the marrow space. Results are good in terms of pain relief, but motion may remain poor, especially if there is associated rotator cuff pathology. The recovery period is long, 3 to 6 months, but typically well tolerated as it is not a weight-bearing joint and patients are allowed ambulation and mobility as they recover. Shoulder replacement surgery is less common than knee and hip replacement surgery since the shoulder is not a weight-bearing joint and tolerates arthritis relatively well.

CONDITIONS THAT AFFECT THE AC JOINT

While the glenohumeral joint enjoys most of the fame, attention, and publicity associated with the shoulder, there exist a few conditions that affect the AC joint as well. Like any joint, the AC joint can develop arthritis, and if the ligaments of the AC joint are injured, it can become unstable. Let's examine the condition of AC joint instability first.

AC Joint Instability (Shoulder Separation)

The AC joint is stabilized by an interesting and unique system of ligaments. The joint has the intracapsular ligaments that most joints have embedded in the walls of their joint capsule, but it also has a remote set of ligaments that stabilize the AC joint by binding the clavicle to the coracoid process. Since the coracoid and the acromion are two parts of the same bone, binding the clavicle to the coracoid stabilizes the AC joint. For some odd reason, dislocations of the AC joint are called shoulder separations (not AC joint dislocations). In these injuries, a traumatic event injures one or more of the AC joint ligaments, destabilizing the joint.

There are seven types of AC joint separations. The lowest-grade AC separation (type I) occurs when the intracapsular ligaments are strained, but not torn. This injury results in pain and tenderness over the AC joint and, if the joint fills with blood, can also result in a mild "bump" deformity. In a type II AC joint separation, the intracapsular ligaments are torn, but the coracoclavicular ligaments remain intact. This results in a more obvious deformity and a greater level of discomfort. If all of the AC ligaments are torn, the deformity and discomfort are even greater. This is known as a type III separation.

Figures 2-47, 2-48, and 2-49 show the ligament injuries, the clinical appearance, and the x-ray findings associated with types I, II, and III AC joint separations, respectively. Type I separations present with pain and a mild deformity but no x-ray changes. Patients with type II separations have clinical findings similar to those with type I separations, but have noticeable displacement of

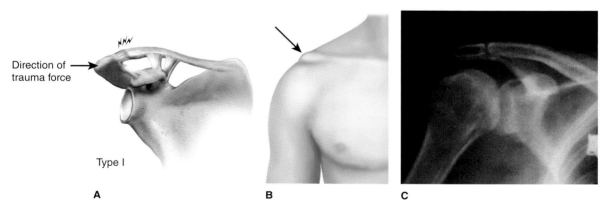

Figure 2-47. The anatomic basis (left), clinical appearance (middle, with arrow pointing to the AC joint deformity), and x-ray findings seen with a type I AC joint separation.

the joint on x-ray. It is common to describe this deformity by saying that "the clavicle is sticking up," but the clavicle is actually right where it belongs. Gravity pulls the rest of the shoulder girdle down, making it appear that the clavicle is up. In the type II AC joint separation, displacement of the AC joint is less than 100%, meaning that a portion of the clavicle is still articulating with the acromion. Type III separations have even greater clinical deformity, and the

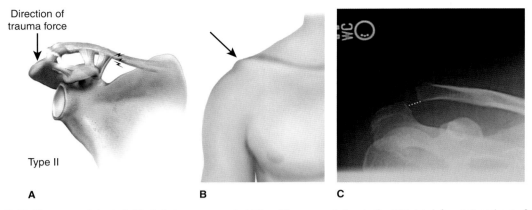

Figure 2-48. The anatomic basis (left), clinical appearance (middle, with arrow pointing to the AC joint deformity), and x-ray findings seen with a type II AC joint separation.

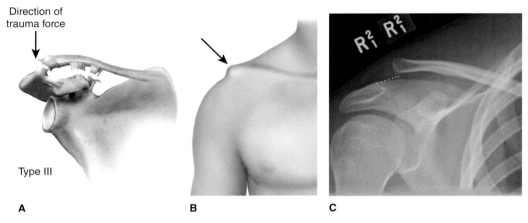

Figure 2-49. The anatomic basis (left), clinical appearance (middle, with arrow pointing to the AC joint deformity), and x-ray findings seen with a type III AC joint separation.

x-ray shows greater than 100% displacement of the joint (no portion of the clavicle articulates with the acromion). In the type III separation, all of the stabilizing ligaments are torn. Types IV, VI, and VII are very rare. A type V separation (Figure 2-50) is just an extreme version of a type III, where the clavicle is protruding through the trapezius muscle and is tenting the skin.

Type V AC joint separations are typically treated surgically, with open ligament reconstruction. Types I and II are treated nonoperatively, with a sling for comfort for 1-4 weeks, depending on the level of discomfort. The treatment of type III dislocations is controversial, with some surgeons advocating operative and others nonoperative treatment. Scar tissue usually forms to provide type III AC joint separations managed conservatively with adequate joint stability, but the "bump" deformity is permanent.

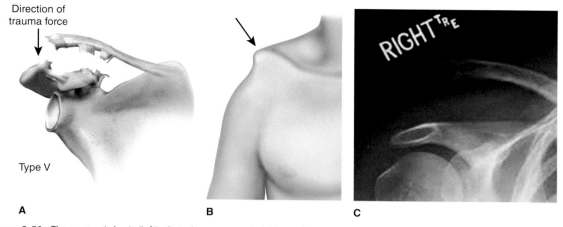

Figure 2-50. The anatomic basis (left), clinical appearance (middle, with arrow pointing to the AC joint deformity), and x-ray findings seen with a type V AC joint separation.

Those treated with open ligament repair trade a bump for a scar. Functional results tend to be excellent in both groups.

AC Joint Arthritis

The AC joint of the shoulder has a range of motion that is much smaller than the glenohumeral joint, but, with time and use, its articular surfaces can become worn and rough, leading to AC joint arthritis (Figure 2-51). Patients with AC joint arthritis are

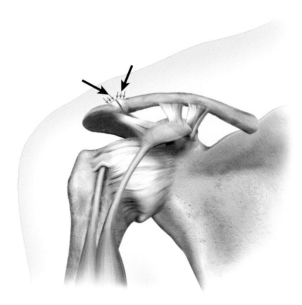

Figure 2-51. A drawing depicting degenerative arthritis of the AC joint (arrows).

easy to differentiate from patients with other shoulder conditions because, on physical examination, palpation over the AC joint (which is easy to find on almost every patient) reproduces their pain. The easiest bone to identify on physical exam is the clavicle. To find the AC joint, "walk" your fingers laterally along the subcutaneous surface of the clavicle until you encounter a small ridge, or bump. This is the AC joint. Tenderness to palpation over the AC joint suggests AC joint arthritis or, if there is a history of trauma, an AC joint separation (see previous discussion). The "cross-arm impingement test" can be used to diagnose AC joint arthritis as well. To perform this test, the patient reaches across their chest to grasp the back of the opposite, asymptomatic shoulder. This position compresses the AC joint, and if it is inflamed, it will reproduce the patient's pain (Figure 2-52).

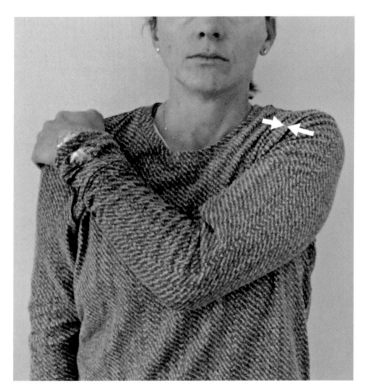

Figure 2-52. The "cross-arm impingement" test can be used to diagnose an inflamed AC joint. Have the patient reach across their body to grasp their contralateral shoulder. This compresses the AC joint and will reproduce the patient's pain if the AC joint is inflamed.

▶ Imaging

Patients with AC joint arthritis will often have osteophytes, joint space narrowing, or small cystic changes on the articular surfaces of the clavicle or acromion that are visible on a standard AP x-ray (Figure 2-53). Be aware, however, these the x-ray findings are relatively common in older, completely asymptomatic patients and are probably only meaningful in patients with a positive physical exam.

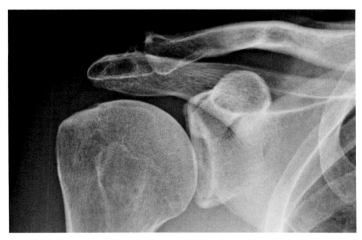

Figure 2-53. An x-ray showing the joint space narrowing, osteophytes, and cystic changes typical of AC joint arthritis.

▶ Medical Treatment

Many times, symptomatic AC joint arthritis can be effectively managed with a short course of NSAIDs and, if that isn't successful, a cortisone injection into the AC joint (see Chapter 9 for a simple, in-office AC joint injection technique). While nonoperative treatments do not correct the pathologic architecture of arthritic AC joint surfaces, they often provide long-term relief to patients who have acute episodes of AC joint arthritic symptoms resulting from overuse or other precipitating activities. Physical therapy has not been shown to be particularly effective in the non-operative management of AC joint arthritis.

▶ Surgical Treatment

The surgical treatment of AC joint arthritis takes advantage of the fact that the joint has a redundant system of stabilizing ligaments. In general, the operations designed to treat arthritic joints employ one of three different strategies: fusion (arthrodesis), resurfacing (arthroplasty), or joint resection (see the sidebar The Three Surgical Treatments for Arthritis in Chapter 4, page 135.) The method that works best for the AC joint is resection. The distal 1 cm of the clavicle is removed (Figure 2-54), leaving a 1-cm gap between the acromion and the distal end of the clavicle. Once the distal piece of clavicle is removed, this gap fills with blood, and this volume of blood hardens and matures into a "plug" of scar tissue that acts

BEWARE OF REFERRED PAIN!

The shoulder is a common target for referred pain from other sources. If you are working with a patient who has shoulder pain and nothing you are trying is working, consider the possibility that your patient's shoulder pain may not be shoulder pain at all. Figure 2-R shows some of the many conditions that

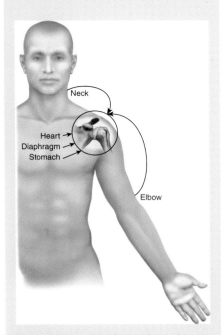

Figure 2-R. Nonshoulder conditions that can present as shoulder pain include myocardial ischemia, lateral epicondylitis of the elbow, and cervical radiculopathies.

are known to refer pain to the shoulder. The one I encounter most frequently is cervical radiculopathy. If your patient is complaining of pain that radiates below the elbow, of numbness or tingling, pain that radiates into the neck, shoulder pain that is made worse with head and neck movements, or pain that is posterior (scapular pain), be suspicious. Shoulder pain with these qualities can be the result of a cervical radiculopathy.

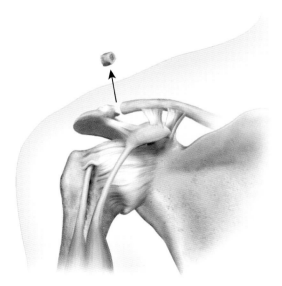

Figure 2-54. Resecting the distal 1 cm of the clavicle is the preferred surgical treatment for AC joint arthritis.

as a cushion between the two bones of the AC joint, eliminating the arthritic pain that occurred when the two bones articulated against each other. The AC joint is particularly well suited for this procedure. Joint resection would be a poor choice for the treatment of knee joint arthritis, for example, since it would result in a radically unstable knee joint. But, the second set of AC joint-stabilizing ligaments, the coracoclavicular ligaments, allows for excellent joint stability, even after the primary set of AC joint ligaments, the ligaments integral to the AC joint capsule, are resected with the distal end of the clavicle. For a review of the system of ligaments that stabilize the AC joint, refer to Figure 2-3.

LABRAL TEARS

As mentioned, there is a dense, thickened portion of the glenohumeral joint capsule along the rim of the glenoid socket. If the labrum (and therefore the capsule) are traumatically separated from the bone of the glenoid rim, this can create glenohumeral joint instability. Remember that the ligaments that stabilize the glenohumeral joint are in the substance of the capsule, so if the capsule is detached from the glenoid, the stabilizing ligaments are detached as well. In the most common type of glenohumeral joint dislocation (the anterior dislocation), it is the anterior/inferior capsule and labrum that become detached. A labral tear in this location is known as a "Bankart tear." Repairing the capsule and labrum back to the glenoid socket rim is an important part of the surgical procedure used to address recurrent shoulder dislocations.

The long-head biceps tendon is another structure that originates from the labrum. It attaches at the twelve o'clock position, and it can pull the labrum off of the socket rim, creating what is called a SLAP (superior labrum, anterior-to-posterior) tear. SLAP tears don't tend to result in instability but can cause pain. SLAP tears are difficult to diagnose. There is no "typical" history for such an injury, and the physical exam tests we have developed so far are not particularly sensitive or specific. Many in the field of orthopedics argue that SLAP tears are clinically irrelevant, while others contend that they are an important source of shoulder pathology. There is no good consensus on what forms of conservative management work best. Most practitioners will start with a program of physical therapy, but it is not clear exactly what therapy program works best. Surgical results, especially the results of operations designed to address type I tears (fraying of the superior labrum) are often unpredictable and sometimes disappointing. All of this makes it difficult to provide clear and concise recommendations regarding how to diagnose and address superior labral tears, if they need to be addressed at all.

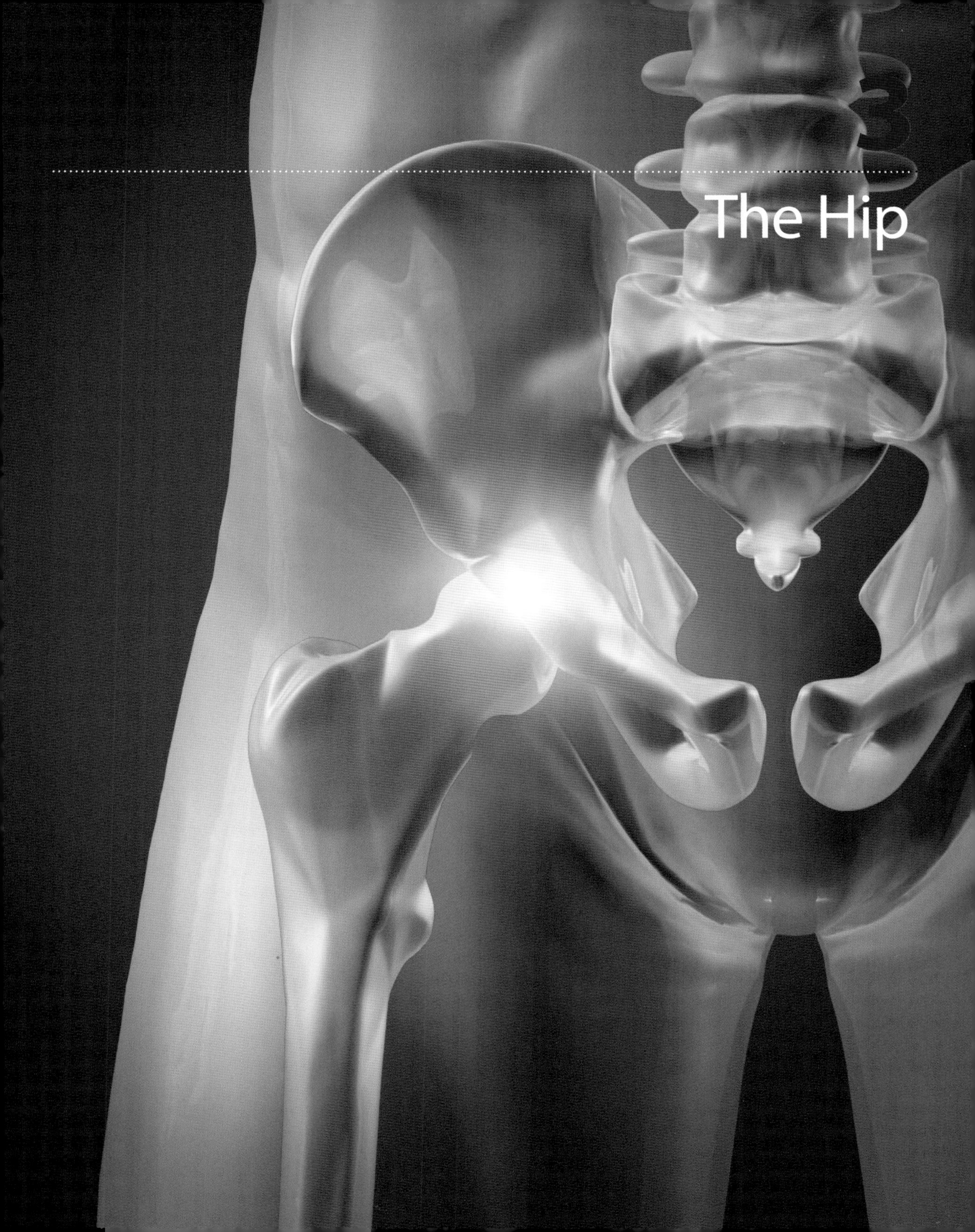

3 The Hip

The differential diagnosis for a patient presenting in an outpatient clinic with hip pain is relatively narrow. It's been said that when you hear hoofbeats, think horses, not zebras. In other words, those hoofbeats you're hearing are more likely to be coming from common things (horses) than uncommon things (zebras). That makes good sense and is practical, but just to be safe, we will cover both the "horses" and the "zebras" in this chapter. The horses (common conditions) are hip arthritis, greater trochanteric bursitis, and hip pain that is actually pain radiating down from the lumbar spine. These three hip conditions account for over 90% of the hip pain you are likely to encounter in an outpatient setting. The occasional patient with avascular necrosis (AVN) or a form of femoral-acetabular impingement (FAI), make up the other 10%—these are the zebras.

HIP ARTHRITIS

Let's start with hip arthritis. As discussed in Chapter 1, in orthopedics, we consider arthritis to be a disease of the articular surfaces of the joint. Figure 3-1 shows a hip joint that has been dislocated to show the head of the femur and acetabular socket better. In a normal

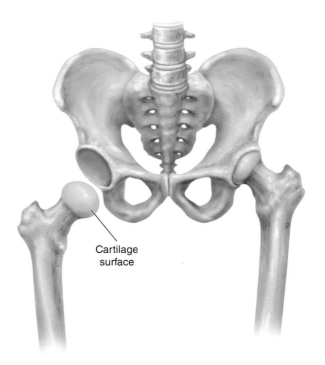

Figure 3-1. The ball and socket of a normal hip joint.

hip, both the surface of the femoral head and the surface of the socket are coated with a 2- to 4-mm thick layer of slick, numb articular cartilage. Most patients are familiar with this material because they have seen it on the ends of chicken bones (see the sidebar in Chapter 1, page 18 for more details). In arthritis, this material wears thin or, in some instances, is gone completely, exposing the underlying bone. Bone is not slick and slippery; it is rough and abrasive. It isn't numb like articular cartilage either. It has a rich nerve supply and, as a result, is very sensitive and a poor bearing surface for a weight-bearing joint. Figure 3-2 shows an arthritic femoral head with a large area of worn cartilage and exposed bone.

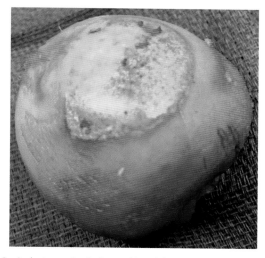

Figure 3-2. A photograph of a femoral head that shows changes typical of arthritis. There is a large area where the articular cartilage has been worn off to expose the rough, abrasive, sensitive bone beneath it.

The most common cause of hip arthritis is osteoarthritis. In osteoarthritis, the articular cartilage simply wears away with time and use. For this reason, most patients with osteoarthritis of the hip are older. A history of "high mileage" is probably the single most important factor in a patient's history that predicts osteoarthritis. High mileage can mean many decades of normal use or a few decades of heavy use. Patients with hip arthritis usually complain of groin pain and will often remark that they have trouble getting their shoes and socks on due to hip pain and stiffness.

▶ Physical Exam

The hip joint capsule (Figure 3-3) is an envelope, or membrane, of firm but flexible tissue that surrounds the joint. It is attached to the

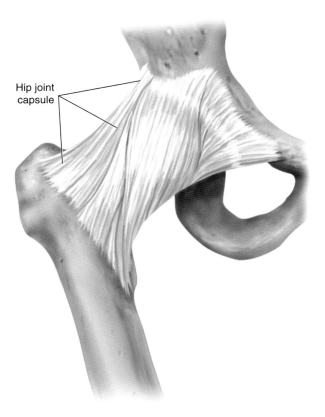

Hip joint
capsule

Figure 3-3. The hip joint capsule, a tough fibrous membrane that envelops the hip joint.

rim of the socket on the acetabular side and the neck of the femur just below the femoral head on the femoral side. Hip joint fluid is contained within the capsule, and the capsule helps hold the ball inside the socket.

When the hip is inflamed, the synovial cells overproduce joint fluid, and the capsule becomes tense and distended. Some of the pain and stiffness that patients with hip arthritis have is from the pressure that develops in the overdistended hip joint capsule. If the hip joint is flexed 90 degrees, as it is when the patient is seated on the exam table, and we internally and externally rotate the femur, we greatly increase the pressure inside the overdistended capsule (sort of like wringing out a washcloth). Typically, the patient will complain of pain, and we will find that the arthritic hip does not rotate as freely or through as great a range of motion as the asymptomatic hip. This physical exam test (internal and external rotation of the hip in 90 degrees of flexion) is called the "windshield wiper test" and is illustrated in Figure 3-4.

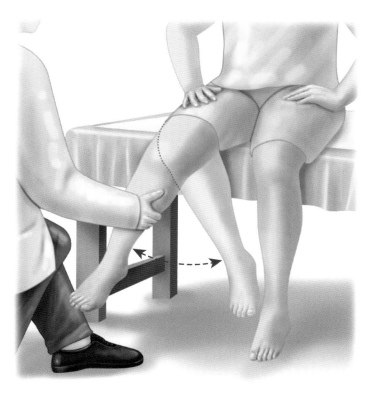

Figure 3-4. The "windshield wiper test" (passive internal and external hip rotation in 90 degrees of flexion). Pain and stiffness suggest hip joint arthritis.

▶ Imaging

The best diagnostic tool for detecting hip arthritis is a plain anteroposterior (AP) pelvis x-ray. Since the cartilage coating on the surface of the ball and socket are invisible on x-ray, a normal hip joint with a healthy layer of articular cartilage surface appears to have a gap between the surface of the ball and the surface of the socket. This gap is sometimes referred to as the *joint space*, but technically speaking, there is no space. The cartilage on the surface of the ball is resting directly on the cartilage surface of the socket; it is just that these surface materials are not visible on the x-ray, so there appears to be a space. Figure 3-5 is an AP pelvis x-ray. The hip on the patient's left (our right) is normal and has no significant narrowing of the apparent joint space. The patient's right hip has lost all of the cartilage on both the femoral head and the acetabular socket in the area marked by the arrow. In this part of the patient's right hip joint, the bone of the ball is resting directly on the bone of the socket. This is what is termed *bone-on-bone* arthritis. Less-advanced cases of hip arthritis will have joint spaces that are narrower than the asymptomatic side but are not yet down to bone on bone.

SEEING ARTHRITIS ON AN X-RAY

The following are the four radiographic signs of arthritis (Figure 3-A):

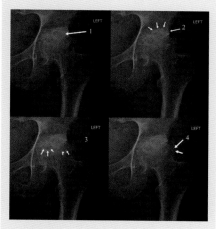

Figure 3-A. An x-ray showing the four radiographic signs of arthritis: (1) narrowing of the apparent joint space, (2) subchondral sclerosis, (3) subchondral cysts, and (4) osteophytes (bone spurs)

1. **Narrowing of the apparent joint space.** The loss of radiolucent articular cartilage narrows the space between the two bones.

(continued on following page)

2. **Subchondral sclerosis.** Bone density increases when bone is subjected to increased forces. Joints with little or no articular cartilage left articulate with greater friction and compression forces, so the bone just beneath the surface of the joint (known as the subchondral bone) becomes more dense and radiopaque.

3. **Subchondral cysts.** Small foci of bone necrosis on the surfaces of arthritic joints create small, lucent lesions known as subchondral cysts.

4. **Osteophytes.** For some reason, perhaps in an attempt to distribute increased joint forces over a larger area, arthritic joints grow extra bone along their articular margins. These "bone spurs" are referred to as *osteophytes*. Because they have a sharp, pointed appearance, patients often believe that these osteophytes are what cause the pain of arthritis, and that, if the bone spurs could be removed, their pain would improve. Unfortunately, surgically removing osteophytes from an arthritic joint has not been shown to significantly decrease joint pain. The pain is more likely the result of direct stimulation of the nerves in the exposed bone surfaces and pain from over distension of the joint capsule, both of which are still present after the osteophytes are removed.

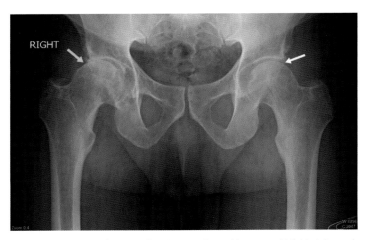

Figure 3-5. An AP pelvis x-ray showing a patient with a normal left hip joint and right hip bone-on-bone arthritis. Note the dark, radiolucent "gap" between the ball and the socket on the healthy left hip (white arrow). The dark space between the ball and the socket is full of healthy cartilage. There is an area where there is no cartilage between the ball and socket of the patient's right hip (yellow arrow).

▶ Medical Treatment

Since a portion of the joint pain and stiffness in an arthritic hip is due to excess fluid within the joint capsule, medications that "deflate" the capsule by decreasing the production of inflammatory fluid tend to help. Nonsteroidal anti-inflammatory drugs (NSAIDs) most likely work in this way. Similarly, an intra-articular cortisone injection may help as well. These injections are usually given using image guidance, and a technique for administering an intra-articular hip cortisone injection is outlined in Chapter 9. Though anecdotal evidence exists to support the use of nutritional supplements (glucosamine, chondroitin sulfate, MSM [methylsulfonylmethane], etc.) to treat arthritis, the results of large, randomized, prospective, blinded trials have not shown these treatments to be effective. Strategies to decrease joint compressive forces include weight loss and the use of assistive devices such as a cane, crutches, or a walker. Physical therapy can help by increasing the flexibility and compliance of the joint capsule, allowing it to accommodate swelling better.

▶ Surgical Treatment

The surgical treatment for hip arthritis is a hip replacement. In this operation, the acetabular socket is resurfaced with a layer of low-friction material (usually polyethylene plastic), and the rough, worn femoral head is replaced with a smooth, polished ball made of either metal or ceramic (Figure 3-6). To secure the ball to the shaft of the femur, the ball is connected to a titanium stem that fits inside the hollow marrow cavity of the femur bone. Early designs were bonded to the bone with bone cement (a technique that is still

---

TWO CRUMMY OPERATIONS ...

Late in the second half of the 19th century, physicians were starting to experiment with the concept of hip joint replacement. At that time, a common

(continued on following page)

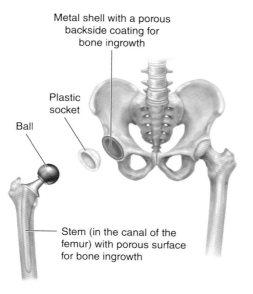

Metal shell with a porous backside coating for bone ingrowth

Plastic socket

Ball

Stem (in the canal of the femur) with porous surface for bone ingrowth

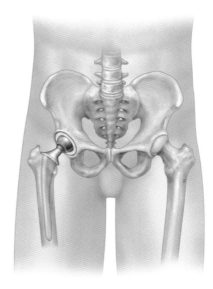

Figure 3-6. The components of a contemporary total hip replacement.

used if the bone is very osteoporotic), but more modern devices have a porous texture on the surfaces of the stem that allows bone to actually grow to the implant. The polyethylene plastic socket is contained in a metal shell that has a similar coating that allows it to bond to the bone of the acetabulum. As an operative procedure, the hip replacement operation has been a tremendous success. Few surgical procedures can match its track record for safety and patient satisfaction.

GREATER TROCHANTERIC BURSITIS

Another common cause of hip pain is greater trochanteric bursitis. Figure 3-7 shows the bony prominences created by the greater trochanters of the proximal femur bones. The greater trochanters are usually palpable on the lateral sides of the hip joints. The iliotibial band (IT band or ITB) originates from the *ilium* of the pelvis and inserts on the lateral *tibia* just below the knee joint. This dense strap of connective tissue is the tendon of the gluteus maximus and tensor fascia lata muscles, and it passes back and forth over the greater trochanter like a windshield wiper when we walk. The relationship between the IT band and the greater trochanter is shown in Figure 3-8. If the IT band becomes too tight and rubs against the trochanter with too much friction, it can cause swelling in the greater trochanteric bursa and create a focus of inflammation known as greater trochanteric bursitis.

procedure was to surgically excise the ball and neck of the arthritic hip, then allow the void to fill with blood, which would later harden into scar tissue and form a dense scar "spacer" between the femur and the acetabulum. The result was what is called a *resection arthroplasty*. The operation was feasible because it was fast. There was no anesthesia at that time, so only short procedures were practical. The operation eliminated the pain from bone grinding against bone in the joint, but the resulting scar articulation wasn't as strong or stable as a normal hip. Innovators in the field started experimenting with materials that could be interposed between the femur and acetabulum. Glass, gold foil, and pig bladder were some of the materials that were used, but none worked well. Figure 3-B shows an x-ray of a resection arthroplasty performed on a patient who had right hip arthritis. Note the "empty socket." The resection arthroplasty operation is also known as a *Girdlestone* procedure.

(continued on following page)

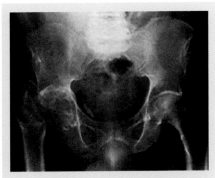

Figure 3-B. An AP pelvis x-ray showing a resection arthroplasty of the right hip. Note that the femoral head has been resected and the socket is empty

The other procedure that was used to treat hip arthritis was called a *hip fusion*, or *arthrodesis*. In this procedure, the raw, exposed bone on the surface of the femur is screwed to the raw, exposed bone on the surface of the socket. As is the case with a fracture, the two exposed bone surfaces will heal together if held still and in close apposition for 6-8 weeks. The result is that the pelvis and femur become one solid bone. Like the resection arthroplasty, this operation eliminated the pain from bone rubbing against bone, and it had the advantage of being more stable. But, the pain relief that this procedure afforded patients came with a price: the joint could no longer move.

HOW LONG WILL IT LAST?

A modern hip replacement is a wonderful operation, with low complication rates and high patient satisfaction scores, but like all human-made devices, the implants will inevitably wear out over time. The components themselves are actually fairly durable. As you would expect, the weakest link in the system, in terms of wear, is the plastic socket liner. But, even these wear relatively slowly.

(continued on following page)

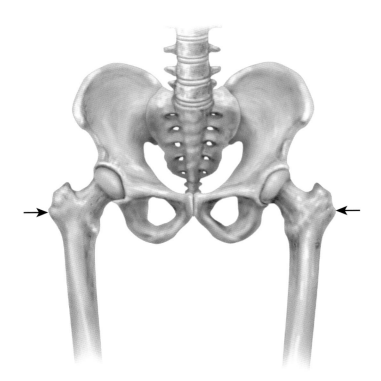

Figure 3-7. The greater trochanters (arrows) are bony prominences on the lateral side of the proximal femur.

Patients with greater trochanteric bursitis usually complain of lateral sided hip pain. The pain is typically worse when they try to sleep on their side at night. If they sleep with their affected side down, the pressure of the mattress on the inflamed bursa bothers them. If they try to sleep with their affected side up, they have pain because, as the up-side thigh drops down across the midline to rest on the down-side thigh, the IT band is stretched to an even greater extent over the trochanter. Patients will often say that the only way that they can sleep comfortably on their sides is to sleep with their affected side up and with a pillow between their knees to keep the tension from developing in the IT band. Rarely, the IT band will catch or snap on the trochanter creating a palpable, or even audible, "clunk." This "clunk" can be so profound that patients with this condition, called *coxa saltans*, are often convinced that their hip is dislocating when this occurs.

▶ *Physical Exam*

Patients with greater trochanteric bursitis will usually have little or no pain or stiffness on the windshield wiper test. They will,

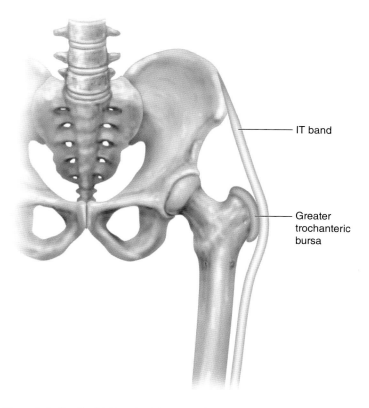

IT band

Greater
trochanteric
bursa

Figure 3-8. The iliotibial band originates on the ilium of the pelvis and inserts on the lateral side of the proximal tibia. It passes back and forth, from anterior to posterior, over the greater trochanter with each cycle of hip joint flexion and extension.

however, be tender to palpation over the greater trochanter (Figure 3-9). When checking for tenderness to palpation over the greater trochanter, be sure to press on the trochanter of the patient's unaffected hip as a control since slight tenderness to palpation over this bony landmark can be positive in patients who don't have trochanteric bursitis. Hip x-rays on patients with greater trochanteric bursitis will be negative, and other studies, such as magnetic resonance imaging (MRI) scans, may show a fluid collection in the greater trochanteric bursa. Typically, the diagnosis of greater trochanteric bursitis can be made by history and physical exam, and no imaging studies are necessary.

▶ Treatment

The first stage of treatment for greater trochanteric bursitis typically consists of IT band stretches and NSAIDs. The stretches are intended to restore flexibility and elasticity to the IT band so that it rubs with less friction against the greater trochanter. One can

The plastic of a modern hip replacement socket wears at a rate of less than a tenth of a millimeter a year. Given that the plastic is usually on the order of a centimeter thick, it would take 100 years for a patient to wear all the way through one. Why is it, then, that our total hip replacements don't last the patient's lifetime?

While a few hip replacements will fail as a result of unusual complications such as infection and dislocation (each accounting for about 1% of total hip failures), most will fail because the bond between the replacement part and the bone fails. Like a crown that comes off of a tooth, the bonded interface between the socket or stem and the bone loosens over time, and when it finally fails, the hip replacement components are no longer affixed to the skeleton, and they move or shift a tiny bit when the patient walks. This motion of the device against the adjacent bone is painful.

One of the factors that can hasten the process of component loosening is *wear debris*. It turns out that, as the ball rubs against the plastic socket liner, the liner sheds tiny, submicron particles of plastic into the joint fluid. These particles are about the same shape and size of bacteria, and they elicit a robust immune reaction. That immune reaction attacks both the plastic particles and the bone/prosthesis interface, and this weakens the bone near the implant, which leads to loosening. Once the association between polyethylene plastic wear debris and component loosening was recognized and confirmed by multiple investigators at multiple institutions, the goal became to limit or eliminate these particles. The "gold standard," a metal ball articulating against a traditional plastic socket liner, generated the highest volumes of polyethylene plastic debris. The first innovation was to strengthen the plastic of the socket liner by a process called cross-linking. This step alone led to an order of magnitude decrease

(continued on following page)

in polyethylene debris. Other bearing surface combinations were also tried. A metal ball articulating with a metal socket liner was attractive because it yielded no plastic particles at all. Unfortunately, the particles that metal on metal bearings shed, cobalt and chromium metal ions, appear to have a toxic affect locally in the hip joint and systemically throughout the body. For this reason, metal-on-metal bearings have fallen out of favor among hip replacement surgeons. Another interesting bearing material is ceramic. Ceramic ball-and-socket liners provide articulations that do not shed any plastic particles. In fact, the ceramic material is so hard, so smooth, and so wear resistant that it is hard to measure any wear debris of any kind in these joints. The problem with ceramics turned out to be chipping, cracking, and fracture, as well as high manufacturing costs. A bearing surface combination that remains an attractive choice, especially in young patients, is a ceramic ball in a cross-linked polyethylene plastic socket liner. Because the ceramic is smoother than metal, a decrease in wear debris of over two orders of magnitude can be achieved when compared to a metal ball in a traditional plastic socket. Because the plastic liner is softer than a ceramic liner, chipping, cracking, and fracturing are less common as well.

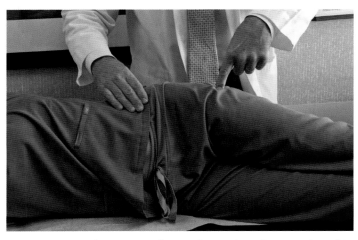

Figure 3-9. To test for greater trochanteric bursitis, have the patient lie on his or her side and press firmly over the greater trochanter (the most prominent palpable bone on the lateral side of the hip joint). Be sure to check the contra-lateral side as a control; a slight amount of tenderness to palpation over the greater trochanter is considered normal. In the photo above, the examiner's left index finger is pressing against the patient's greater trochanter.

write a physical therapy prescription for IT band stretches and tensor fascia lata/gluteal muscle eccentric strengthening exercises, or the patient can simply do a set of home IT band stretches on their own. The popular home stretches for the IT band are the supine crossover stretch (Figure 3-10) and the standing wall stretch

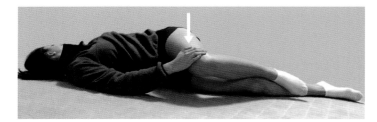

Figure 3-10. The supine crossover stretch for the IT band. The patient lies on his or her back. The side to be stretched is laid across the midline and as close to the floor as possible.

(Figure 3-11). The home stretches should be done for 30 seconds to a minute 10 times a day for 3 to 4 weeks. Oral anti-inflammatory medications help by decreasing inflammation in the bursa. If a program of NSAIDs and stretches doesn't succeed, a greater trochanteric bursa cortisone injection can be safe and effective. A technique for administering a greater trochanteric cortisone injection is outlined in Chapter 9. There are no good surgical solutions for greater trochanteric bursitis. In fact, operating in this area can

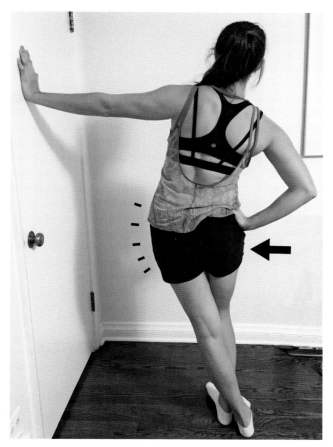

Figure 3-11. The standing wall stretch for the IT band. The patient stands with their hand against the wall. The IT band of the hip closest to the wall is stretched by crossing the foot of that leg behind the other foot and pushing the pelvis toward the wall.

create scar tissue in the ilio-tibial band, which can make it less flexible and make the condition worse.

LUMBAR SPINE PATHOLOGY

Hip arthritis and greater trochanteric bursitis constitute two of the three common causes of hip pain seen in an outpatient setting. The third common cause is low back pain that radiates into the hip, buttock, or thigh. Symptoms that strongly suggest that a patient's hip pain is coming from their spine include pain that radiates below the knee, numbness and tingling, especially if it radiates down into the foot or toes, and pain that radiates below the hip into the posterior thigh. On physical examination, these patients will have normal, pain-free range of motion on the windshield wiper test and no greater trochanteric tenderness. They may

HIP JOINT DISLOCATIONS

One of the potential complications of total hip replacement surgery is dislocation (Figure 3-C). A natural hip has a

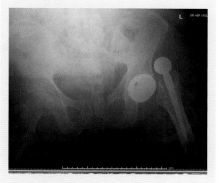

Figure 3-C. A dislocated total hip joint

strong but flexible ligament connecting the ball to the socket of the joint. This ligament, the ligamentum teres, prevents the ball from coming out of the socket (see Figure 3-15). Though a few designs have been considered, no hip replacement has ever been manufactured with a connector like this. Metal chains and cables scratch the bearing surfaces of the ball and socket, and other, softer materials aren't durable enough. We have had to omit this important ligament, and, as a result, human-made hip joints are inherently more prone to dislocating than mother nature's original design. Fortunately, dislocation is an infrequent complication of artificial hips, occurring in only about 1% of patients.

WHAT'S THE BEST WAY TO GET THERE?

If you are planning to climb a mountain peak, you must first choose a route. Chances are, several routes to the top of that peak exist, each with their own advantages and disadvantages, and every so often, an innovative thinker will discover a clever new route that no one else has thought of. The same is true regarding the surgical approach used to perform a total hip replacement. We can approach the hip joint from the back (a posterior approach), the side (a lateral approach), or the front (a direct anterior approach). All of these approaches can be used to get the job done, and all have been used successfully in legions of patients, but the direct anterior approach is gaining widespread popularity because fewer muscles are injured in this approach, resulting in faster healing times and shorter hospital stays.

LOSING YOUR HEAD: WHY IS THE FEMORAL HEAD PRONE TO AVASCULAR NECROSIS?

It is tempting to think of bone as an inanimate frame onto which our living organs and tissues are attached, but bone is just as much a living tissue as any other tissue in the body, and, as such, it requires a blood supply to survive. Bones are designed to have a limited blood supply. To be strong, they have thick, dense cortical walls that would be structurally weakened if they had tunnels and channels coursing through them to accommodate a network of blood vessels. While there is some limited degree of blood supply that comes from the marrow cavity inside the

(continued on following page)

have radicular findings (decreased sensation, motor weakness, or reflex changes). An AP pelvis x-ray will show normal hip joint anatomy but may show degenerative changes in the lower lumbar spine, which is often visible on the AP pelvis x-ray.

There are many patients who have both hip arthritis and an element of hip pain that comes from lumbar spine pathology. The challenge then becomes determining how much of their pain is coming from each location. Using a series of differential cortisone injections can help sort this out. If you are struggling to sort out where the hip pain in your patient is coming from, you may want to administer an intra-articular hip joint injection, a lumbar epidural injection, and even a hip trochanteric bursa injection, each spaced 2 weeks apart, and use the results to determine which location is responsible for the patient's symptoms. Techniques describing how to administer these injections can be found in Chapter 9.

THE ZEBRAS … LESS-COMMON CAUSES OF HIP PAIN

If you can diagnose hip arthritis, greater trochanteric bursitis, and hip pain that is actually radiating down from the lumbar spine, you will be well equipped to handle most of the patients with hip pain that you will encounter in an outpatient practice. But, there are a few less-common conditions that can cause hip pain symptoms, and two of these are worth covering here.

Avascular Necrosis

The head of the femur is particularly vulnerable to ischemia (see sidebar). Due to peculiarities in the shape and size of the blood vessels that nourish the femoral head, these vessels are relatively easy to occlude. If these vessels become occluded, the bone in the center of the head can die. This creates a weak spot within the substance of the head, and with weight-bearing forces, the ball can collapse (Figure 3-12). Early in the disease, radiographic findings may be subtle. Figure 3-13 shows an x-ray typical of AVN. Patchy areas of density and lucency are seen within the femoral head; if you look closely on this example, you also can see a "step-off" on the surface of the ball indicating early collapse, as well as fragmentation of the femoral head bone.

In its early stages, AVN can be hard to see on an x-ray. An MRI can be more useful in detecting early AVN. Figure 3-14 shows the dramatic signal changes seen in the femoral head typical of AVN. In more advanced cases of AVN, the head collapses and the ball flattens, and the resulting shape mismatch between the ball and the socket dramatically increases the wear rate of articular surfaces, leading to arthritis.

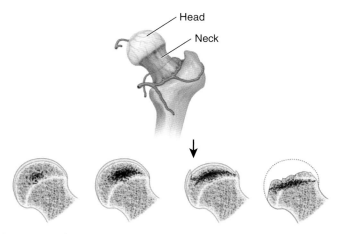

Figure 3-12. The blood vessels that nourish the femoral head are small and follow a circuitous path. They are prone to occlusion if blood viscosity is increased, causing the bone in the center of the head to die, which can lead to femoral head collapse.

▶ Physical Exam

The windshield wiper test is typically positive in patients with AVN, especially in the later stages when the femoral head collapses and joint congruity is lost.

▶ Treatment

There is no proven medical treatment for AVN of the femoral head. By the time it is diagnosed, it is too late to initiate any treatment that might decrease blood viscosity in an attempt to increase blood flow to the femoral head. Fortunately, the disease has a limited clinical course, and the necrotic lesion in the femoral head eventually heals. Approximately one-third of patients heal their lesion without

bone (called the *endosteal* blood supply), the principal blood supply comes from a few blood vessels that insert onto the surface of the bone (called the *periosteal* blood supply). Delivering blood to the femoral head is a particularly challenging problem, since the vast majority of the head is covered with cartilage and therefore "off limits" for blood vessel insertion. No blood vessels can attach to this bearing surface. The blood vessels that nourish the head have to take a circuitous path *within* the bone to reach their destination. There is a single vessel that travels in the substance of the ligamentum teres and inserts at the apex of the femoral head, but this vessel is rarely patent in adults. Most of the blood supply comes from vessels in the femoral neck. These are small-caliber vessels that are branches of the femoral circumflex arteries. They have to make a "U-turn" to enter the femoral neck, then take a long trip up the neck to arrive at their destination in the femoral head. Because these are small-diameter vessels taking multiple twists and turns, any condition that increases blood viscosity can occlude them. Though the fine details of the pathophysiology of AVN remain

(continued on following page)

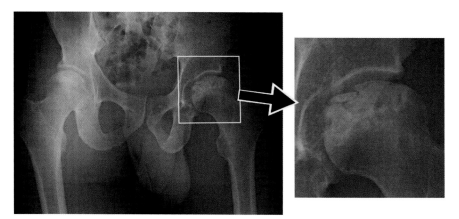

Figure 3-13. An x-ray showing an example of AVN of the femoral head. Note the "step-off" on the articular surface of the ball and fragmentation of the femoral head.

unknown, it does appear that AVN results from occlusion of these small vessels, resulting in the death of the bone in the femoral head. Conditions such as sickle cell disease and Gaucher disease increase the viscosity of blood and can cause AVN. Systemic corticosteroid administration can cause the white blood cells that line the walls of blood vessels to enter the bloodstream and increase blood viscosity. This process, called demargination, is thought to be responsible for the link between corticosteroid use and AVN of the hip. Alcoholism has been linked to AVN as well, perhaps because of fat emboli that result from fatty liver changes.

This same analysis explains why children who become bacteremic will occasionally develop septic arthritis of the hip joint. There is a relative stasis of blood flow in these small-caliber vessels. If there are bacteria in the bloodstream, they will tend to leave the blood and enter tissue in locations where blood flow is slowest. It is analogous to sediment in a river. The sediment will precipitate out of the water in places where the rate of flow is slowest.

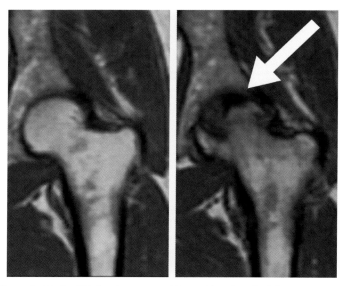

Figure 3-14. An MRI showing a normal femoral head on the left image, with uniform white (fat) signal throughout. The image on the right shows a hip with AVN. The femoral head signal is heterogeneous, with patchy areas of light and dark indicating zones of varying degrees of bone death (arrow).

any collapse or change in the geometry of the femoral head. The other two thirds will also heal, but only after the head has collapsed and the joint is ruined. So, the goal of treatment is to allow the disease to run its course and heal without femoral head collapse.

One option for treatment is to ask the patient to use crutches or a walker for 6 weeks to 3 months. If the joint is not under compressive forces, the chances for collapse are small, and the disease usually runs its course in 6-12 weeks. Another option is a surgical procedure called *core decompression*. In this operation, a small-diameter drill bit is passed into the center of a necrotic lesion under fluoroscopic guidance. Having a core decompression turns the tables on the odds for developing femoral head collapse. Two-thirds of patients with AVN who undergo the procedure *do not* progress to collapse; one-third do. Factors like continuing use of high-dose oral or intravenous corticosteroids make the prognosis worse. Since the sole purpose of the operation is to try to prevent femoral head collapse, the procedure only makes sense in patients who have early AVN and have not yet had femoral head collapse. If the head has collapsed, a hip replacement is the best solution.

Labral Tears and Femoral Acetabular Impingement

Another less-common source of hip pain is impingement between the proximal femur and the acetabulum. The hip joint labrum is a rubbery ring of tissue that sits on the rim of the acetabular socket

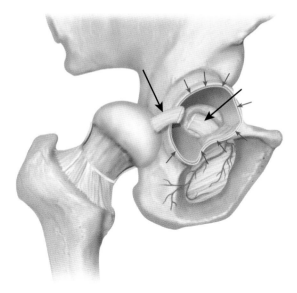

Figure 3-15. The black arrows show the ligamentum teres (the ligament has been divided in this drawing to allow the femoral head to be dislocated out of the acetabulum). The ligamentum teres is a strong ligament that holds the femoral head in the socket. Hip replacements don't have this ligament, so they can dislocate easier than a natural hip. The smaller, blue arrows show the labrum, a thick ring of cartilage on the rim of the acetabulum.

(Figure 3-15). Viewed in cross section, from above, the labrum appears as a small triangle-shaped piece of tissue on the edge of the socket rim (Figure 3-16). Figure 3-17 shows the concave

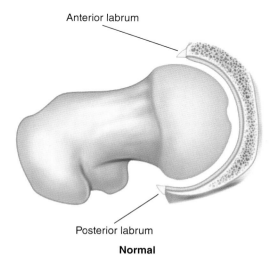

Anterior labrum

Posterior labrum

Normal

Figure 3-16. A cross section of the hip joint as viewed from above, with a cross-sectional view of the anterior and posterior labrum on the rim of the socket.

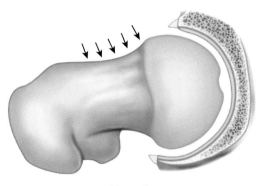

Normal

Figure 3-17. The normal "hourglass"-shaped femoral neck. Note that the surface of the neck is concave (arrows).

contour of the femoral neck (arrows), and Figure 3-18 shows how the edge of the socket and labrum fit into this concavity when the hip is flexed and internally rotated. There is a morphologic variant of the femoral neck known as the "cam-shaped" femur, in which

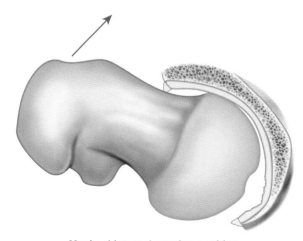

Maximal internal rotation position

Figure 3-18. In certain positions of hip joint rotation, the acetabular labrum comes to rest in the concavity of the femoral neck.

this area of the femoral neck is actually a prominence instead of a shallow valley. Figures 3-19 and 3-20 show a drawing and an x-ray of a cam-shaped femoral neck, respectively; Figure 3-21 shows how a cam-shaped femoral neck can impinge against the rim of the acetabulum, damaging the labrum or detaching it from the bone of the socket rim when the hip is flexed and rotated. Figure 3-22 is an

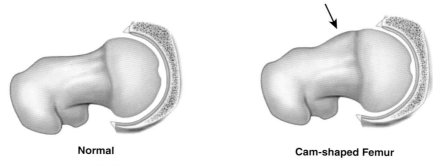

Normal   **Cam-shaped Femur**

Figure 3-19. The anatomic variant of the femoral neck known as the "cam-shaped femur" in which the femoral neck is a hump or mound instead of a shallow valley.

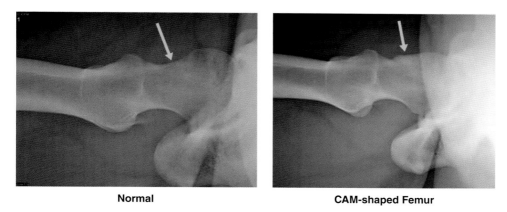

Normal   **CAM-shaped Femur**

Figure 3-20. X-ray examples of normal versus cam-shaped femoral neck anatomy (arrows).

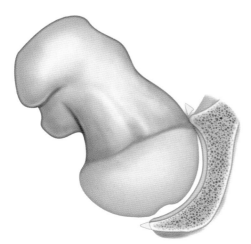

Figure 3-21. In the cam-shaped femur, the extra bone on the surface of the femoral neck can impinge against the labrum, causing the phenomenon known as *femoral acetabular impingement* (FAI). Over time, repeated FAI can tear the labrum and detach it from the rim of the socket.

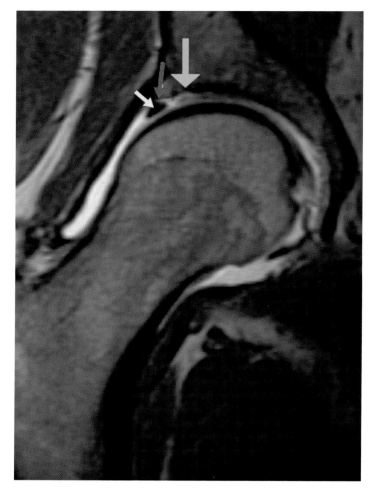

Figure 3-22. An MRI taken after a volume of gadolinium contrast has been injected into the hip joint (this test is called an MRI arthrogram) showing a detached labrum. Note the white colored gadolinium dye (red arrow) in between the bone of the rim of the acetabular socket (yellow arrow) and the detached labrum (white arrow) (*Reproduced with permission from Brian White, MD*).

MRI image of a hip in which the joint has been injected with gadolinium dye. The dye appears white on the image. The study shows that there is dye (red arrow) in between the labrum (white arrow) and the rim of the socket (yellow arrow). This finding indicates that the labrum has become detached, most likely from repeated impingement against the femur.

▶ *Making the Diagnosis*

Diagnosing FAI and labral tears based on history and physical exam can be challenging. There may be a history of trauma or no injury at all. Certain sports, like dancing, gymnastics, and ice skating, seem to make patients particularly prone to this condition. On physical exam, the windshield wiper test will likely reveal pain with combined flexion and rotation, but this finding is not particularly specific and can be absent. In most office settings, this becomes a diagnosis of exclusion: If a patient has hip pain, especially groin pain, no trochanteric tenderness, and the windshield wiper test reproduces their pain *but* plain films show no significant arthritis, one should consider AVN or FAI.

▶ Treatment

Physical therapy, NSAIDs, and image-guided cortisone injections can all play a role in the treatment of FAI and labral injuries. If these conservative treatments are not successful, then surgical intervention can be considered. The extra bone on the neck of the femur can be removed arthroscopically (Figure 3-23) and the

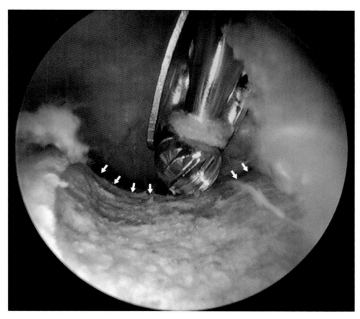

Figure 3-23. An arthroscopic photograph showing the metal tool that is used to grind away the "hump" of excess bone typical of cam-shaped femoral necks. The arrows show an area where the neck has been sculpted down to have a more concave shape (*Reproduced with permission from Brian White, MD*).

labrum repaired back to the rim of the acetabulum (Figure 3-24). If the labrum is too damaged and is not repairable, a soft tissue graft can be installed to reconstruct the labrum.

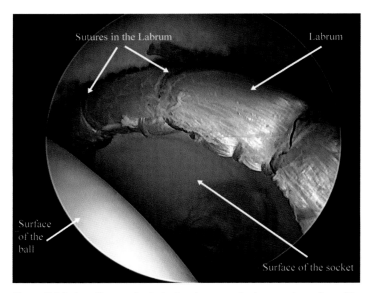

Figure 3-24. An arthroscopic photo showing several sutures and a graft used to reconstruct the damaged labrum on the rim of the hip joint socket (*Reproduced with permission from Brian White, MD*).

Summary

A practical approach for evaluating patients with hip pain is outlined in Figure 3-25. The first step is to evaluate hip joint irritability by applying the windshield wiper physical exam test. If it is positive, then the patient either has arthritis or a zebra such as FAI, a labral tear, or AVN, and a simple x-ray can be used determine if it is arthritis. If the windshield wiper test is negative, test for trochanteric bursitis by checking for tenderness to palpation over the greater trochanter on the physical exam. If there is no tenderness over the trochanter, they either have hip pain emanating from a lumbar spine condition, or one of the unusual zebra conditions.

HIP FRACTURES

A thorough discussion of hip fractures is somewhat out of place in a textbook dedicated to the practice of *office* orthopedics. It is unlikely you will ever encounter a patient who presents with this diagnosis in an outpatient setting. But, as long as our ability to live longer outpaces our ability to reverse osteoporosis, hip fractures will be a growing part of all of our practices. Since the care and management of patients with a hip fracture requires more cooperation and collaboration between medical and orthopedic providers than any other condition we will cover in this text, it seems appropriate to discuss this topic here.

The term *hip fracture* is an inaccurate one. We use the word *fracture* to describe an injury to bone. We talk about radius

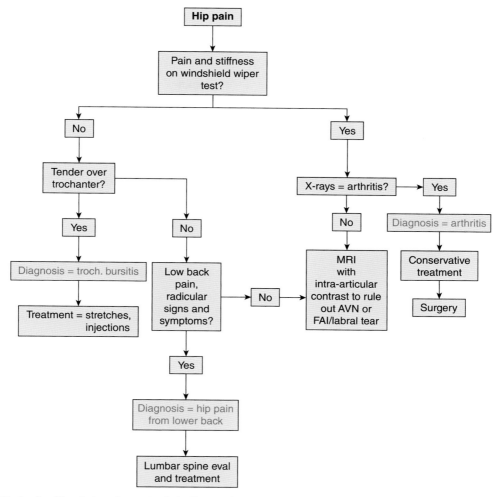

Figure 3-25. An algorithm that can be used to help diagnose in an outpatient setting the conditions that cause hip pain.

fractures, clavicle fractures, and tibia fractures, for example. There is no "hip bone." The hip is a joint between the proximal femur and the pelvis. One would think that fractures of either the ball of the femur or the acetabular socket of the pelvis would be considered hip fractures, but that isn't the case. Fracture of neither of them is considered a hip fracture. By convention, acetabular fractures and all other fractures of the pelvis are *not* considered hip fractures, and femoral head fractures (though they would technically qualify as hip fractures) are rarer than hen's teeth.

So, what exactly *is* a hip fracture? In orthopedics, we consider hip fractures to be fractures of the proximal femur, and over 90% of those occur at one of two anatomic locations: the neck of the femur or the section of proximal femur that lies between the lesser and greater trochanters (Figure 3-26). From

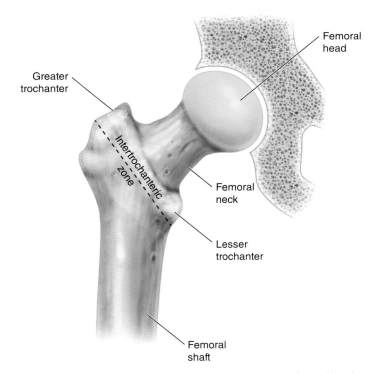

Figure 3-26. The anatomy of the proximal femur showing the femoral head, neck, intertrochanteric zone, and proximal femoral shaft.

an engineering standpoint, this makes sense. If you think about snapping a stick in your hands, it is very hard to get the stick to break a few millimeters from the tip. This would be analogous to breaking the femur through the femoral head. Bending and torsional forces at the head are low. Furthermore, the femoral head is contained within, and protected by, the acetabular socket. As a result of these factors, fractures of the femoral head are very, very rare.

The thinnest, most fragile part of the entire femur bone is the neck. The femoral neck is the short, hourglass-shaped section of bone that joins the ball to the shaft of the femur. The type of hip fracture that occurs here is called a femoral neck fracture, and femoral neck fractures are very common. The other common fracture is called an intertrochanteric fracture. Although the bone between the trochanters is thick and strong, this area is at the apex of the angle between the femoral neck and shaft, and simple physics predicts that this is a weak spot and a place where fractures will occur. Subtrochanteric fractures (fractures that occur just below the lesser trochanter) exist but are relatively rare. Fractures even farther down the femur are called femoral shaft fractures, and these are not considered hip fractures.

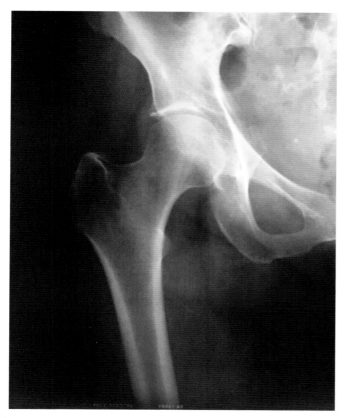

Figure 3-27. An x-ray of a normal right hip joint. Can you see the anatomic features depicted in Figure 3-26?

Figure 3-26 shows the anatomic features of the proximal femur. Can you find all of them on Figure 3-27, a plain x-ray of a normal hip joint? As is the case in Figure 3-27, the greater trochanter is often hard to see. The x-ray technologists are trained to adjust the x-tray beam to be intense enough to image deep structures like the femoral head, which is buried under many layers of soft tissue. An x-ray beam of that level of intensity often overexposes the greater trochanter, which is closer to the surface and is surrounded by less tissue. Figure 3-28 shows the appearance of the two common types of hip fractures: the intertrochanteric fracture and the femoral neck fracture.

▶ Treatment: Surgery

Unlike most orthopedic conditions, there is rarely an indication for the nonoperative management of hip fractures. Before the introduction of hip fracture surgery, a hip fracture in an elderly patient had a greater than 50% mortality rate. It wasn't the injury that was so lethal, it was the treatment, which, at that time, was a period

YOU SAY YOU WANT TO DO WHAT TO GRANDMA!?!

Decreasing mortality and restoring the ability to ambulate are two of the main reasons to treat hip fractures surgically, and hip fracture operations are typically

(continued on following page)

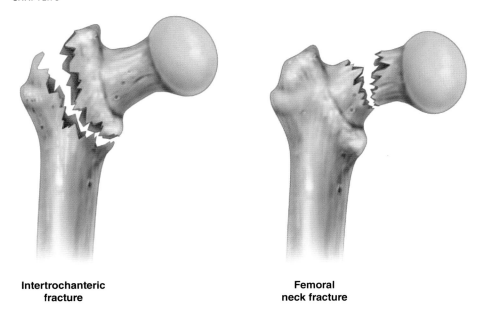

Intertrochanteric fracture   **Femoral neck fracture**

Figure 3-28. The two common types of hip fractures: intertrochanteric and femoral neck.

successful at achieving both of these goals. But, imagine you are asked to see a patient with a hip fracture who has a history of chronic, severe, end-stage dementia. Imagine that the patient doesn't communicate or ambulate, and that this patient has been languishing in a nursing home somewhere for years before falling out of bed and sustaining this injury. For such a patient, a procedure intended to prolong life may not align with the desires of the patient's family, and restoring the ability to ambulate is not possible. Is a major operation still the right choice? In many cases, believe it or not, it is!

I encountered such a patient early in my career. When I suggested to the patient's family that we take Grandma to the operating room for an hour or two of major surgery to fix her hip, they thought I was insane. They explained to me that they were confident that, if Grandma were able to assess her current condition, she would not choose to prolong her life. They refused to consent to the surgery

(continued on following page)

of 6 weeks to 3 months of bed rest. A protracted period of strict bed rest in older patients who often had preexisting comorbidities such as heart disease, respiratory compromise, and poor peripheral circulation resulted in all of the complications we associate with prolonged immobilization. Deep vein thrombosis, pulmonary embolism, pneumonia, aspiration, and pressure ulcers were common, and these and other complications often started a downward spiral that culminated in the death of the patient. The surgical solutions invented to treat hip fractures decreased mortality to closer to 10% because these treatments allowed earlier mobilization of these medically frail patients. In addition to decreasing the mortality rates associated with hip fractures, hip fracture surgery increased the chances that the patient would regain the ability to ambulate. A loss of the ability to ambulate has been correlated with poor outcomes in elderly patients. A third benefit of hip fracture surgery is pain management. It is difficult to provide patients with a hip fracture with adequate perineal care, log rolling, and other nursing essentials due to the pain of an untreated hip fracture (see sidebar).

For all of these reasons, surgery is usually the treatment of choice for patients with hip fractures. What is interesting is that the type of surgery is so different for these two different types of hip fractures, fractures of the same bone that occur within an inch or two of each other. Intertrochanteric fractures are treated with an *osteosynthesis* operation, a procedure that uses metal plates, screws, or rods to join the fracture fragments together so that the fracture will heal. Femoral neck fractures, when displaced, are treated differently. These fractures are typically treated with hip replacement surgery.

The reason for the difference is related to the blood supply to the femoral head (see Figure 3-12). Displaced femoral neck fractures destroy the blood vessels that nourish the femoral head. These vessels lie in the femoral neck and are interrupted by femoral neck fractures. This results in the death of the femoral head through the process of AVN. The dead femoral head eventually dissolves, leaving only the femoral neck in the acetabular socket. Osteosynthesis operations don't work for most displaced femoral neck fractures because the dead femoral head won't heal to the proximal femur, no matter how well the two bones are fastened together surgically.

For that reason, the operation of choice is to remove the dead femoral head and replace it with one made of metal. Often, the acetabular side of the joint is normal and does not need to be replaced. Since only half of the joint is being replaced (just the ball, not the ball *and* socket), this operation is *half* of a total hip, so it is called a *hemiarthroplasty*. Bipolar hip replacements and fixed-head endoprostheses are types of hemiarthroplasties used to treat displaced femoral neck fractures. A standard total hip replacement that includes a socket replacement component is used if the patient happens to have significant hip joint arthritis as well as a displaced femoral neck fracture, and mounting evidence seems to indicate that pain relief may be superior when the socket is replaced as part of the operation. Performing a total hip replacement (as opposed to a hemiarthroplasty) is a longer and more costly operation, so the risks and benefits of treating patients with a total hip versus a hemiarthroplasty have to be considered. Figure 3-29 shows the

I proposed, and she went back to the nursing home for palliative care. About 3 weeks later, I received a call from the family explaining that they had changed their minds. Grandmother wasn't tolerating bed rest well. She had been having episodes of bad diarrhea, and the nurses were having a hard time taking care of her. They wanted to know if it was too late for her to have her hip fixed. When she came back into the hospital, she was noted to have a down-to-bone sacral ulcer. It appeared that the sacrum itself was infected. The surgical solution to her particular fracture was a hip replacement, but I could not implant such a device given her large, infected, open wound and sacral osteomyelitis. She was treated with a diverting colostomy to keep fecal material away from her sacral ulcer, and she underwent a plastic surgery procedure to move a flap of gluteal muscle over the area of exposed sacral bone. The pressure ulcer eventually healed, but the patient passed away before getting the hip replaced.

(continued on following page)

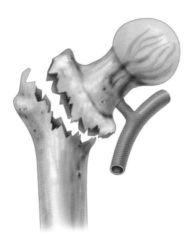
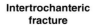
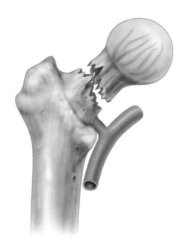

Intertrochanteric fracture   **Displaced femoral neck fracture**

Figure 3-29. A drawing showing how the blood supply to the femoral head is preserved in an intertrochanteric fracture and interrupted in a displaced femoral neck fracture.

This patient's clinical course was the exact opposite of what the family wanted. Their grandmother spent the last few months of her life in the hospital and in pain. Early surgical intervention would have stabilized the fracture, decreased her pain, and allowed logrolling, perineal care, and other nursing necessities. This case emphasizes an important indication for the surgical treatment of hip fractures: pain control. If nonoperative care is chosen, pain management needs to be *very* aggressive, and the complications of high-dose narcotics (aspiration, constipation) and the complications of prolonged bed rest (skin breakdown, deep vein thromboses, pneumonia, etc.) should be understood and expected.

two common types of hip fractures and how the blood supply is preserved in intertrochanteric fractures but interrupted by the fracture in displaced femoral neck fractures. Figure 3-30 shows an

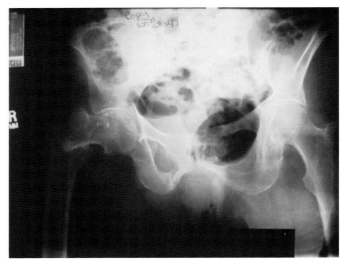

Figure 3-30. An x-ray showing an intertrochanteric fracture of the patient's right hip.

x-ray of an intertrochanteric hip fracture, and Figure 3-31 shows an x-ray of a displaced femoral neck fracture. Figure 3-32 shows an x-ray from the patient discussed in the sidebar on page 109.

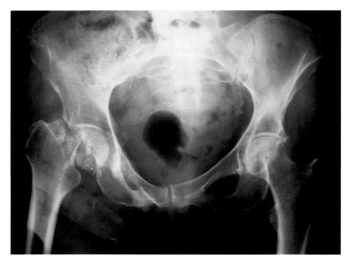

Figure 3-31. An x-ray showing a displaced femoral neck fracture of the patient's right hip.

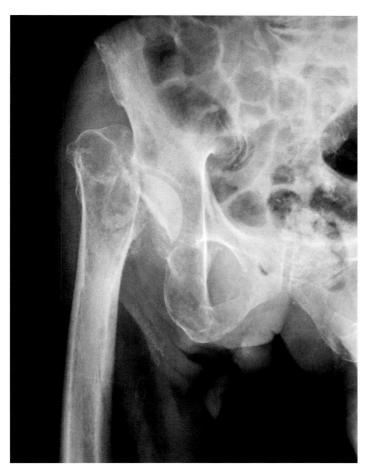

Figure 3-32. An x-ray taken weeks after an untreated displaced femoral neck fracture of the patient's right hip. Note that this fracture has disrupted the blood supply to the femoral head, and the femoral head has almost completely dissolved.

This x-ray shows how the femoral head, which has died from having its blood vessels divided by a displaced femoral neck fracture, dissolves over time.

There is a third type of hip fracture: the nondisplaced, or stable-impacted, femoral neck fracture. In these fractures, there is a fracture through the femoral neck, but it is not displaced enough to damage the blood vessels that nourish the femoral head. In this type of femoral neck fracture, the head will likely survive and can be attached to the proximal femur using an osteosynthesis operation. Typically, three small-diameter screws or pins are used. This operation is called a *hip pinning*. Figure 3-33 shows a minimally displaced, impacted fracture of the patient's right femoral neck. This fracture was treated with a hip-pinning operation. Figure 3-34

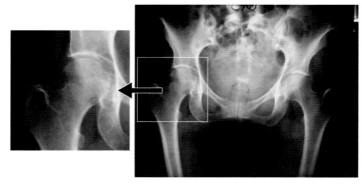

Figure 3-33. An impacted, minimally displaced femoral neck fracture of the patient's right hip. The fracture is subtle, and not easy to see, but if you look carefully, you will see that the hourglass shape of the femoral neck is disrupted, the ball looks like a scoop of ice cream falling off the ice cream cone *(Licensed from Shutterstock)*.

is a 6-month postoperative film of this same patient showing the three screws used to stabilize the fracture and that the fracture has healed.

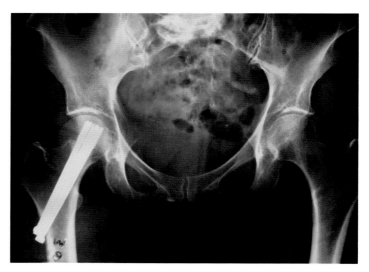

Figure 3-34. The fracture in Figure 3-33 after a hip-pinning operation and subsequent healing of the femoral neck fracture. Nondisplaced, impacted femoral neck fractures have the potential to heal because the vessels that nourish the femoral head remain intact.

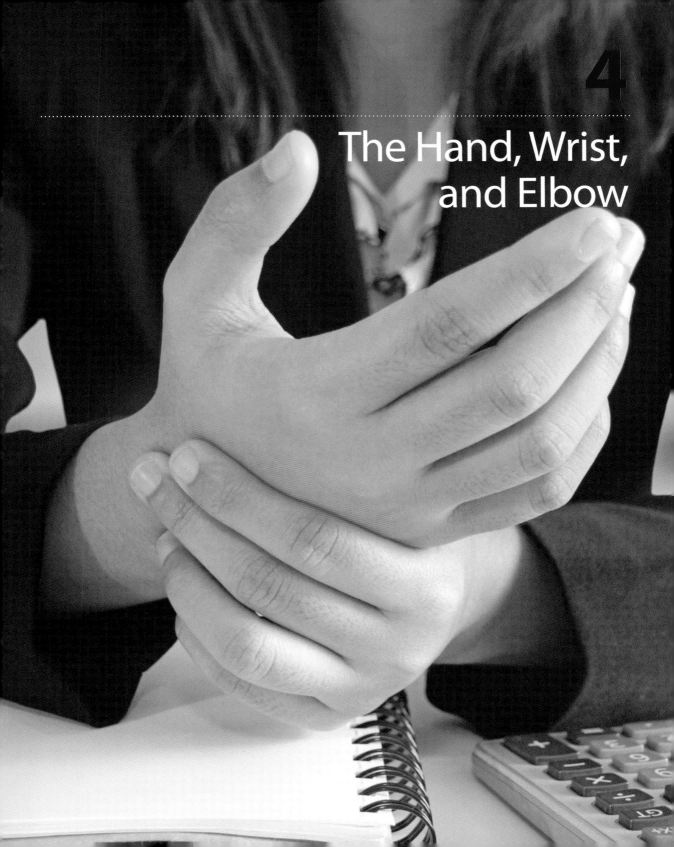

4

The Hand, Wrist, and Elbow

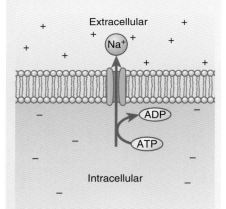
CARPAL TUNNEL SYNDROME

The best way to understand carpal tunnel syndrome is to start by understanding the carpal tunnel. As its name implies, it is an actual tunnel, with a floor, two walls, and a roof. The carpal bones of the wrist make up the floor and both walls of the carpal tunnel, and the roof is a tough, rigid sheet of connective tissue called the *transverse carpal ligament*. The tunnel is 2-4 cm long, and 10 structures travel through it to get from the forearm to the hand: nine flexor tendons and the median nerve (Figure 4-1).

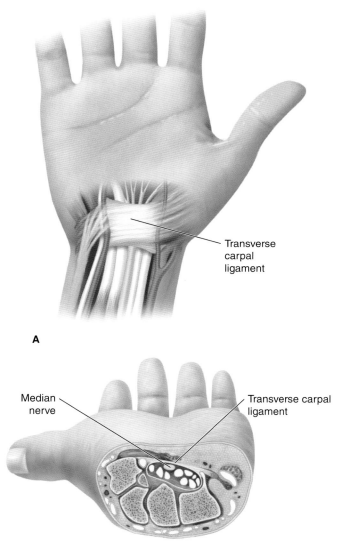

Figure 4-1. A. The transverse carpal ligament. **B.** The carpal tunnel.

Although the flexor tendons and median nerve look similar (long, slender, rope-like tissues), they could not be more different physiologically (see sidebar). The biggest difference is their ability to tolerate ischemia. To operate properly, nerve tissue needs a healthy blood supply. In carpal tunnel syndrome, increased pressures in the carpal tunnel resulting from swelling and inflammation compress the nerve and decrease blood flow to its axons and their hungry, ATP-burning transmembrane ion pumps. Without an adequate blood supply to fuel these pumps, the nerve starts to malfunction, resulting in numbness, tingling, and paresthesias (see sidebar, page 116). As you would predict, these symptoms should only appear in the tissues serviced by the median nerve, which classically include the palm side of the thumb, index, and middle fingers, as well as the lateral side of the ring finger, though some person-to-person variation in this pattern exists (Figure 4-2).

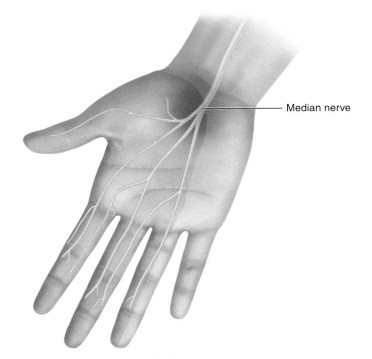

— Median nerve

Figure 4-2. The median nerve distribution.

Neurologic symptoms in other distributions about the hand are likely NOT carpal tunnel syndrome (Box 4-1). Unfortunately, it is rare for patients to offer a precise history of symptoms in the exact median nerve distribution. It can be hard for them to discern/remember the exact distribution of their symptoms when they are giving their history.

A fraction of a second later, all of these mousetraps need to be reset, a job for the ATP-driven transmembrane pumps. Running these pumps 24/7 is an expensive proposition. It requires a great deal of energy, which requires a rich blood supply, and that blood supply can be compromised by pressure. (Press your thumb firmly into your palm. The skin blanches because the pressure drives the blood out of the tissue. Release your thumb, and the skin turns pink again as the blood flow normalizes.) Pressure on the carpal tunnel compromises blood flow in the small vessels that nourish the axons of the median nerve. Under even transient ischemic conditions, the transmembrane pumps run out of fuel and quit working. The nerve starts to malfunction, which we perceive as numbness, tingling, and paresthesias. Most of us have experienced this firsthand. If you sit too long on the hard edge of a toilet seat, your leg will go numb from pressure and local ischemia as your sciatic nerve is pinched between the toilet seat and your femur bone. Relieve the pressure and sensation returns to normal.

Question: What tissue in the human body is *least* sensitive to ischemia?

Answer: Connective tissue, specifically cartilage, ligaments, and tendons.

Tendons are like cables. They are built for strength. Their job is to attach our muscles to our bones and to transmit muscle forces to bone. To keep them strong, they are essentially pure collagen, with very few cells and very few blood vessels in them. The few cells that do exist in tendon tissue (chondrocytes and specialized fibroblasts) are the most metabolically thrifty cells in the human body. They are used to living in ridiculously harsh conditions, exposed to the stress and strain of extreme mechanical forces and the metabolic stress of a severely hypoxic environment. How tough are these connective tissue cells?

(continued on following page)

Viable chondrocytes can be harvested from a person's body days, even weeks, after the person has died!

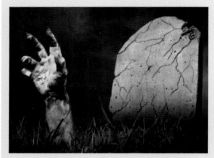

Figure 4-B. *"Night of the living chondrocyte!"* (*Licensed from Shutterstock*)

Box 4-1. Carpal Tunnel Syndrome Is NOT:

- Wrist pain (arthritis?)
- Glove-like distribution of symptoms (neuropathy?)
- Symptoms on the dorsal side of the hand (radial nerve issue?)
- Symptoms in the small and ring fingers (ulnar nerve issue?)
- Symptoms that radiate up the arm (cervical radiculopathy?)

▶ *Physical Exam*

In their history, we expect these patients to complain of numbness, tingling, and paresthesias *in the median nerve distribution.* There are also physical exam findings we can expect. An ischemic median nerve in the carpal tunnel has an unstable axon membrane potential, which we can depolarize by tapping on the nerve. This test, done by tapping over the palmer surface of the carpal tunnel, is called Tinel's sign, and it is considered positive if tapping there produces numbness and tingling in the median nerve distribution. The other two provocative tests are done by increasing pressure in the carpal tunnel, either by pressing firmly onto the transverse carpal ligament (median nerve compression test) or by "kinking" the tunnel by bending the wrist (Phalen's test, Figure 4-3). To better understand

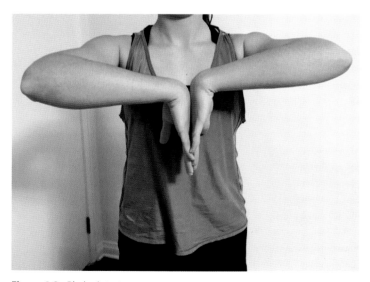

Figure 4-3. Phalen's test.

how Phalen's test works, roll a sheet of paper into a tube, then bend the tube 90 degrees. The "kink" that you create in the paper tube when you bend it demonstrates how Phalen's test compromises the dimensions of the carpal tunnel. When Phalen's test is positive, the patient

increases the volume of the carpal tunnel, taking pressure off the median nerve, and restoring blood flow through the small vessels that nourish the nerve, allowing it to function properly again.

ULNAR NERVE ENTRAPMENT (CUBITAL TUNNEL SYNDROME)

Ulnar nerve entrapment at the elbow (cubital tunnel syndrome) is similar to carpal tunnel syndrome, but it involves the compression of a different nerve (the ulnar nerve) in a different location (the cubital tunnel of the elbow) (see sidebar). The ulnar nerve enjoys a relatively free and comfortable journey from its origins in the brachial plexus in the neck and shoulder area all the way to its most distal innervation targets: the tips of the ring and small fingers. The narrowest, or tightest, section along this pathway is the place where it rounds the corner of the elbow. Here, the ulnar nerve passes through the 2- to 3-inch long cubital tunnel, the floor and walls of which are the humerus and ulna bones and the roof of which is a dense, firm sheet of connective tissue (Figure 4-8).

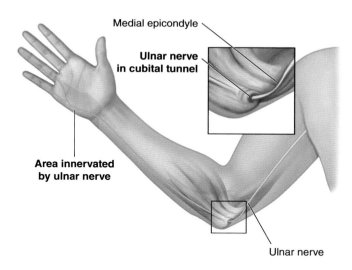

Medial epicondyle

Ulnar nerve in cubital tunnel

Area innervated by ulnar nerve

Ulnar nerve

Figure 4-8. The ulnar nerve at the elbow.

Inflammation in this area can cause compression of the ulnar nerve, resulting in pain, numbness, tingling, and paresthesias in the small and ring fingers. A patient with a history of these complaints could also have a C8 or T1 cervical radiculopathy, thoracic outlet syndrome, or ulnar nerve compression at the wrist, but the most common cause of this pattern of neurologic symptoms is cubital tunnel syndrome.

THE "SQUEEZE ZONE" CONCEPT

Cubital tunnel syndrome and carpal tunnel syndrome (see previous section) both illustrate conditions in which nerve dysfunction results from peripheral nerve axon compression. The mechanism and physiology of this phenomenon are detailed in the sidebar in the section on carpal tunnel syndrome. It is important to understand that for nerve compression to occur, the nerve has to be fixed against some unyielding structure. In carpal tunnel syndrome, it is the carpal bones and the transverse carpal ligament. In cubital tunnel syndrome, it is the medial epicondyle of the humerus, the olecranon process of the ulna bone, and the fascia. The axons of our peripheral nerves travel many inches, often several feet, as they span the distance between their origins (the cell bodies in the spinal cord) to their destinations, for example, the tips of our fingers or toes. Most of that distance is "free and clear," surrounded by soft, flexible fat and muscle. Rarely, there will be a short section along the pathway of the nerve where the nerve passes through a rigid space, such as the carpal tunnel in the wrist or the cubital tunnel in the elbow. Other examples include the area on the lateral side of the knee where the peroneal nerve is tethered to the proximal head of the fibula bone, and the arcade of Froshe where the radial nerve can be trapped by a rigid band of connective tissue in the proximal forearm. These are areas where nerve compression can occur. Any other place along the path of the nerve, the nerve is free to move aside if something tries to push against it. If you hold a garden hose up in the air with one hand and push against it with

(continued on following page)

the other, it just moves away and the water continues to flow. However, if you stand on a hose that is lying on the sidewalk, it will collapse (compress), and the flow through the hose will decrease to a trickle. Mass effects from inflamed tissue, a hematoma, an intervertebral disk (in the case of the spine) are not likely to cause nerve compression *unless* they happen to be pressing against the nerve at a place where the nerve is not free to move out of the way.

▶ Physical Exam

In patients with ulnar nerve entrapment at the elbow, tapping over the cubital tunnel (Tinel's sign) will often create an electrical, shooting sensation into the ring and small fingers, but beware, this test can be positive in normal, asymptomatic patients. If it is negative, and you still suspect cubital tunnel syndrome, I recommend proceeding with conservative treatment. If the patient does not improve, then consider ordering an EMG. Chronic cases may demonstrate wasting of the interosseous muscles of the hand.

▶ Special Studies

Electrodiagnostic studies (EMGs, nerve conduction studies) can be helpful in distinguishing cubital tunnel syndrome from a cervical radiculopathy, thoracic outlet syndrome, or ulnar nerve entrapment at the wrist. When positive, these studies will show a slowing in ulnar nerve conduction across the cubital tunnel.

▶ Medical Treatment

Often, the ulnar nerve is compressed by local inflammatory changes in the cubital tunnel; therefore, NSAIDs can sometimes help. Another useful treatment option is an elbow pad (Figure 4-9).

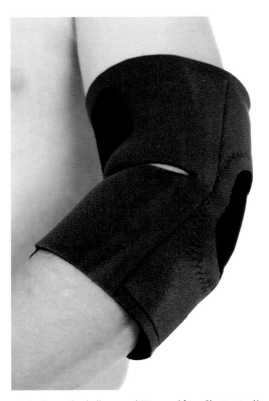

Figure 4-9. A standard elbow pad (*Licensed from Shutterstock*).

The bony prominences around the elbow are common sites of minor contusions in daily life, and those contusions contribute to inflammation. Resting the medial side of the elbow on the hard surface of a desk or table, or the armrest of a car can inflame the cubital tunnel. The elbow pad affords some protection against these everyday occurrences. It also bunches up when the elbow is flexed, limiting elbow flexion and the stretch the ulnar nerve experiences in the cubital tunnel when the elbow is put in the deep flexion position. Patients who have symptoms at night when they sleep with their elbows in the deep flexed position can feel relief by wearing an elbow pad at night.

▶ Surgical Treatment

In cases that do not respond to conservative management, surgery can also be an option. In the most commonly used surgery for cubital tunnel syndrome, the nerve is transposed (moved) out of the cubital tunnel and repositioned more toward the center of the antecubital fossa (Figure 4-10). By "taking a shortcut" across

PHYSIOLOGY OF RECOVERY AFTER NERVE DECOMPRESSION SURGERY

For any nerve decompression surgery, recovery can take months. Some of the axons may have died from nerve compression, and those axons will have to grow back down the length of the nerve to reach their innervation targets. This process, called Wallerian degeneration and regeneration, typically occurs at a rate of a millimeter a day (about an inch of axon growth a month). For that reason, results tend to be better for decompressing nerves that have a short distance to regenerate (such as the median nerve in the carpal tunnel) than nerves that have longer distances (such as the ulnar nerve in the cubital tunnel).

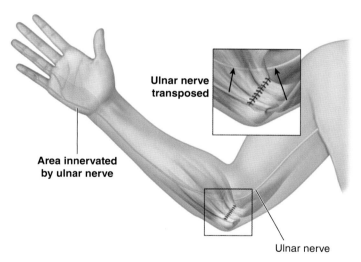

Ulnar nerve transposed

Area innervated by ulnar nerve

Ulnar nerve

Figure 4-10. The ulnar nerve transposition surgery.

the corner of the elbow, there is less tension on the ulnar nerve, especially in deep flexion, and the nerve is freed from the firm, unyielding confines of the cubital tunnel (Figure 4-10 inset). Like most surgical procedures, surgery is indicated if conservative treatment fails. The surgical results of cubital tunnel surgery are not as good as they are for carpal tunnel release. Resolution of symptoms takes longer and is less likely to occur in this operation (see sidebar).

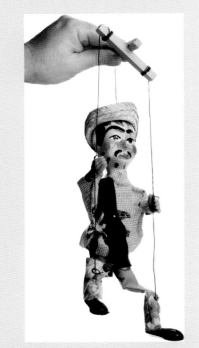

Figure 4-C. (*Licensed from Shutterstock*).

If you ever have the opportunity to look at the bleeding stump of a freshly amputated finger (I have!), you will notice something interesting: We have no muscles in our fingers! (Figure 4-D) Try this:

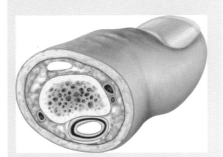

Figure 4-D. Finger (cross section).

(continued on following page)

TRIGGER FINGER

A trigger finger is a finger that becomes stuck in the flexed position. While any finger (or thumb) can have this condition, it is most common in the ring finger. Patients usually report that if they make a fist, then try to straighten their fingers, all of the fingers straighten but one. That finger remains flexed until the patient forces it to extend, which it does with a snap or clunk. If you've ever seen a patient with this condition, it is quite impressive.

▶ *Physical Exam*

There are two physical exam features that are classic for this condition. One is triggering (described above and illustrated in Figure 4-11), and the other is a tender, palpable nodule on the

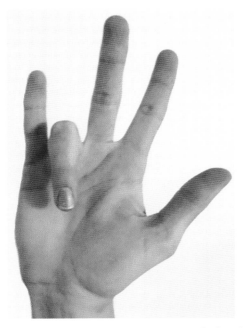

Figure 4-11. Trigger finger: the finger becomes stuck in the flexed position.

palm just proximal to the metacarpal-phalangeal flexion crease (Figure 4-12).

▶ *Medical Treatment*

Trigger finger can often be successfully treated nonoperatively. The goal of treatment is to address the inflammation that creates the flexor tendon nodule (see sidebar for explanation). NSAIDs can help. An extension splint is also an option (Figure 4-13). Bracing the finger in extension eliminates the friction between the

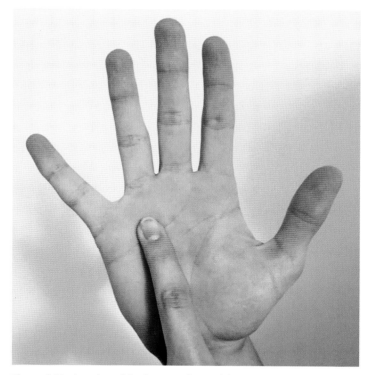

Figure 4-12. Location of the flexor tendon nodule.

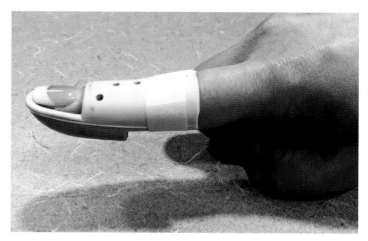

Figure 4-13. A finger splint like this one can be used to treat trigger finger.

tendon nodule and the A1 pulley (see sidebar), allowing the swollen nodule to resolve, eliminating the snag. Another option is a cortisone shot. This is probably the most efficient way to eliminate the inflamed flexor tendon nodule (learn this simple injection technique in Chapter 9).

Roll up your shirt sleeve and turn your hand palm up. Wiggle your fingers wildly. See all of the muscles moving in your forearm? All of the muscles that move our fingers are in our palms and forearms. None of them are in our fingers. This is a great design. If the muscles that moved our fingers were in our fingers, our fingers would be thick and bulky, and that would limit us from doing delicate, fine motor tasks that require thin, nimble digits.

The forearm and hand muscles that operate our fingers are connected to them remotely by long, string-like tendons (put your hand out in front of you with your wrist cocked up and your fingers spread wide, like you would do if you were signaling "STOP." That's the best way to see and appreciate the extensor tendons just beneath the skin on the back of your hand). These tendons are like the strings on a string puppet, moving the fingers remotely.

Look at this schematic drawing of a lateral view of a finger showing the flexor and extensor tendons (Figure 4-E).

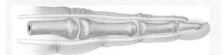

Figure 4-E. Finger tendon schematic.

There is an extensor tendon on the dorsal surface of the finger and an opposing flexor tendon on the palmer surface. To flex the finger, we pull on the flexor tendon.

To extend the finger, we pull on the extensor tendon (Figure 4-F). On the flexor side of the finger, the tendon passes through a series of hoops that function like the eyelets on a fishing rod (Figure 4-G).

These are called the annular and cruciform pulleys. The purpose of the flexor tendon pulleys is to keep the tendon from "bowing" out away from the bones when the tendon is flexed. In the trigger

(continued on following page)

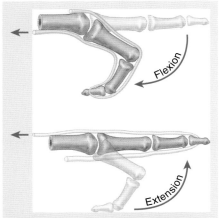

Figure 4-F. Tendons flexing and extending the finger.

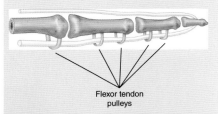

Figure 4-G. Finger tendon pulleys.

finger condition, the patient develops an inflamed, swollen nodule on the flexor tendon that catches as the tendon tries to pass through one of the pulleys. Typically, the nodule catches on the most proximal pulley, which is called the A1 (for first annular) pulley. The more the nodule catches on the pulley, the more inflamed and swollen it becomes, which leads to more catching, which leads to more swelling, which leads to more catching, and so on (Figures 4-H and 4-I).

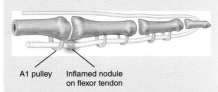

Figure 4-H. The flexor tendon nodule and A1 pulley.

(continued on following page)

▶ *Surgical Treatment*

The surgical solution to trigger finger is safe, simple, and effective, but it is different from what you might predict. Understanding the mechanism of the trigger finger condition (explained in the sidebar), you might expect that the operation would be to "whittle down" the tendon nodule (Figure 4-14). If we do this, it does

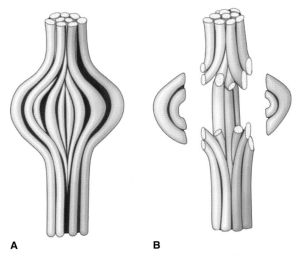

A   **B**

Figure 4-14. A bad idea: debriding the flexor tendon nodule.

eliminate the flexor tendon nodule, but it severs too many of the load-bearing fibers in the substance of the tendon, and tendon rupture is likely to result. Instead, what is done is to divide the A1 pulley (Figure 4-15A). The edges of the divided pulley "pop" open,

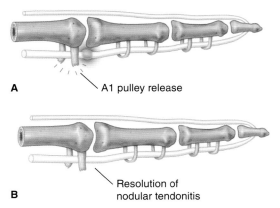

Figure 4-15. A schematic drawing of the finger with its flexor and extensor tendons and the system of pulleys which hold the flexor tendon close to the bones. In this drawing, the most proximal (A1) pulley has been released to relieve catching of an inflamed flexor tendon nodule (trigger finger). B shows that after the A1 pulley is released, the flexor tendon nodule resolves.

and there is no longer friction between the flexor tendon and the pulley. Without a pulley to get stuck on, the tendon glides freely, and the triggering phenomenon is gone. In the absence of friction, the inflamed tendon nodule resolves as well (Figure 4-15B).

THUMB PAIN

Thumb pain is a commonly encountered complaint in any medical office that cares for musculoskeletal conditions. Fortunately, the differential diagnosis for thumb pain is very narrow. Most patients suffer from either DeQuervain syndrome or arthritis of the joint at the base of the thumb (the first carpal-metacarpal [1st CMC] joint). A traumatic source of thumb pain that you may see in your office is an injury to the ulnar collateral ligament of the thumb metacarpal-phalangeal joint, also known as skier's thumb or gamekeeper's thumb.

DeQuervain Syndrome

DeQuervain syndrome is a tendonitis that occurs on the dorsal side of the wrist near the base of the thumb (see sidebar). The location of the pain may lead us to confuse it with 1st CMC joint arthritis, but using a few simple tests, we can differentiate between these common conditions. DeQuervain syndrome is a tendonitis (sometimes called a *tenosynovitis*) of the two tendons that share the first extensor compartment tendon sheath on the dorsum of the wrist. This sheath is like a hollow straw that the tendons pass through as they travel beneath a tight band called the extensor retinaculum (Figure 4-16). As the tendons slide back and forth in the sheath, they can rub against the sharp distal edge of the extensor retinaculum, creating friction and inflammation in the tendon sheath. Patients complain of pain on the thumb side of the wrist that may radiate up the thumb side of the distal forearm.

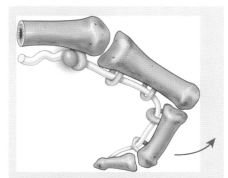

Figure 4-I. A finger "triggering." The nodule on the flexor tendon becomes caught under the A1 pulley, locking the finger in the flexed position.

THE ANATOMIC SNUFFBOX

DeQuervain syndrome is an inflammatory tendonitis of the two tendons that reside in the first extensor tendon sheath (the abductor pollicis longus and the extensor pollicis brevis). There are five extensor tendon sheaths on the dorsal side of the wrist, starting with the first on the thumb (radial) side of the wrist and ending with the fifth on the pinky (ulnar) side of the wrist. The second extensor tendon sheath is hard to appreciate on physical exam. It contains the two radial side wrist joint extensor tendons (extensor carpi radialis longus and extensor carpi radialis brevis), but its neighbors, the first and third extensor tendon sheaths, are easy to feel, and often even *see* on physical exam. They create the borders of a hollow dimple, or soft spot, known as the *anatomic snuffbox* (Figure 4-J). The radial (lateral-most) extensor tendon sheath is the first. Using the anatomic snuffbox to help you locate the first extensor tendon sheath is key when giving a cortisone injection for DeQuervain syndrome (learn this technique in Chapter 9). Another valuable use of the anatomic snuff box in orthopedics has to do with scaphoid fractures. Patients with wrist injuries who

(continued on following page)

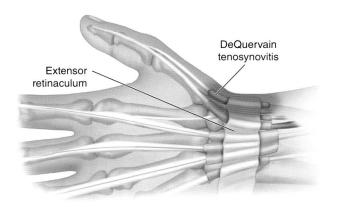

Figure 4-16. The extensor tendon sheaths on the dorsum of the wrist.

Extensor retinaculum

DeQuervain tenosynovitis

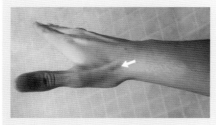

Figure 4-J. The anatomic snuffbox.

are tender to palpation over the anatomic snuffbox may have sustained a fracture of the scaphoid bone. Scaphoid fractures can be difficult to diagnose and, if missed, can lead to a wrist instability pattern that results in premature degenerative wrist arthritis (see Chapter 8).

For some reason, this condition is particularly common in post-partum women.

▶ *Physical Exam*

There is a very sensitive and specific physical exam test for DeQuervain syndrome, and it has a funny name: Finklestein's test. To perform the test, ask the patient to put their thumb in their palm, then wrap their fingers around their thumb to make a fist with their thumb tucked inside, then have them tilt their wrist toward their pinky finger (Figure 4-17). If they have DeQuervain syndrome, this will re-create their pain, and usually the patient's pain response to this test is dramatic.

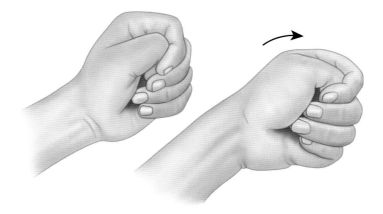

A

B

Figure 4-17. Finklestein's test.

▶ *Medical Treatment*

Often, a few weeks in a brace that immobilizes the wrist and thumb (called a thumb spica splint, Figure 4-18) will cure the condition.

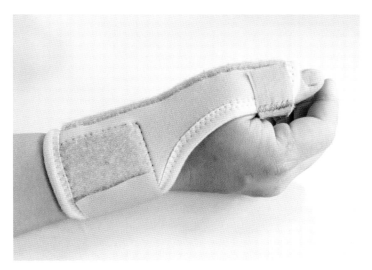

Figure 4-18. The thumb spica splint (*Licensed from Shutterstock*).

If symptoms persist, a cortisone shot into the first extensor tendon sheath is almost always curative (to learn this simple injection technique, refer to Chapter 9).

▶ *Surgical Treatment*

The surgical treatment for DeQuervain syndrome is to release the sheath around the tendons. It is typically effective, but rarely used since cortisone injections work so well.

Arthritis at the Base of the Thumb (AKA basal joint arthritis, 1st CMC arthritis, trapeziometacarpal joint arthritis)

Few joints in the hand work harder than the 1st CMC joint (Figure 4-19). Unlike the finger joints, which essentially work like simple hinges, the joint at the base of the thumb pivots in almost every direction. The muscle forces are greater here, too. Look at the palm of your hand. That big wad of muscle on the thumb side of your palm (the thenar eminence) allows the thumb to exert high forces in many different positions. With all of this force and motion occurring here, it is no wonder that this joint wears out more frequently than all the joints around it.

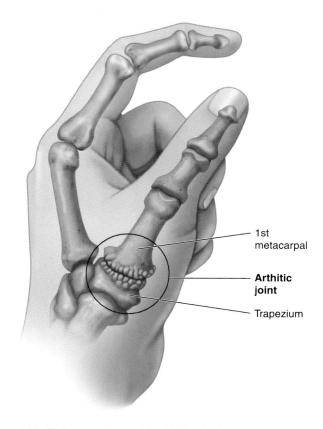

Figure 4-19. First carpometacarpal (1st CMC) arthritis.

▶ Physical Exam

The *CMC grind test* is the test designed to detect 1st CMC arthritis. To perform the test, hold the patient's palm in one hand and their thumb in the other. Compress the 1st CMC joint by pushing the thumb into the hand and, while holding that compressive force, rotate the thumb in a big circle (Figure 4-20). As you move the thumb, think of how you would use a mortar and pestle to grind up peppercorns (Figure 4-21). This motion will likely reproduce the pain in a patient with 1st CMC joint arthritis.

▶ X-rays

A simple anteroposterior (AP) and lateral view x-ray of the thumb can help in making the diagnosis. Patients with 1st CMC arthritis will have a loss of apparent joint space between the first metacarpal and the trapezium bone (Figure 4-22). Beware, however: Many older, asymptomatic patients have radiographic evidence of arthritis at the 1st CMC joint.

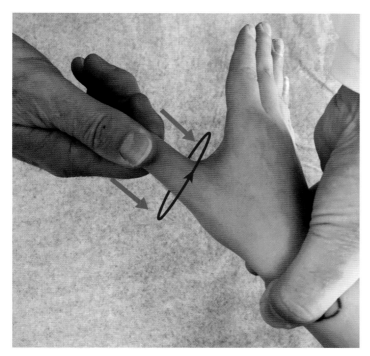

Figure 4-20. First carpometacarpal (1st CMC) grind test.

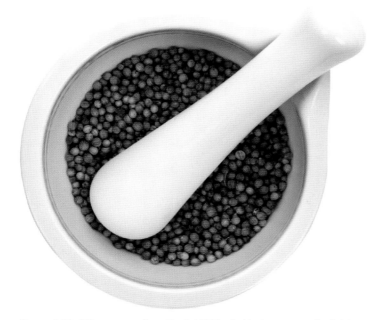

Figure 4-21. When you perform the 1st CMC grind test, compress the joint and rotate thumb metacarpal. It's the same motion you would use when using a mortar and pestle *(Licensed from Shutterstock).*

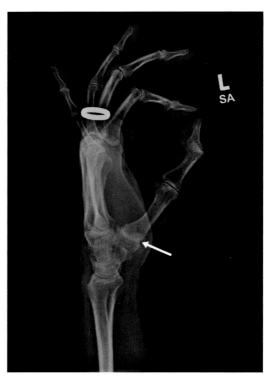

Figure 4-22. An x-ray showing arthritis of the 1st CMC joint at the base of the thumb. Note that there is no joint space between the thumb metacarpal and trapezium bones, indicating a "bone-on-bone" articulation.

▶ *Medical Treatment*

In many cases, 1st CMC arthritis can be treated nonoperatively. A 1- to 2-week period of immobilization in a wrist brace that immobilizes the thumb (called a thumb spica splint) can help relieve the pain of an acute exacerbation. There is also a simple physical therapy exercise that patients can try on their own at home: Place a sponge in a bucket or pail filled with warm water. Place the bucket near a sink. Once the sponge is saturated with warm water, take it out of the bucket and hold it over the sink. Gently squeeze the water out of the sponge and into the sink. Repeat this exercise until all of the water has been transferred from the bucket to the sink. The warmth and motion can help relieve the pain from any arthritic condition that affects the hand or fingers, including 1st CMC arthritis. Some will suggest patients squeeze or knead putty, but the sponge is softer than putty, and patients doing the bucket exercise also receive the benefit of the warmth of the water. Many patients find good and long-lasting relief from cortisone injections into the 1st CMC joint. A simple and effective technique for administering a 1st CMC cortisone injection is covered in Chapter 9.

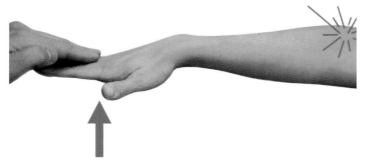

Figure 4-27. The resisted extension test for lateral epicondylitis. The patient's elbow, wrist and fingers are held out straight in full extension. The patient presses up against the resistance of the examiner's hand. The test for medial epicondylitis is the exact opposite: palm up, the patient flexes the out-stretched fingers and wrist against resistance.

resistance should re-create the pain in a patient with *lateral epicon-dylitis*. The elbow, wrist, and fingers should all be straight out in full extension for this test. This starting position stretches, and thus pre-loads, the extensor muscle groups. Pain over the *medial* epicondyle with resisted finger and wrist *flexion* suggests *medial epicondylitis*. Be sure to do both the tests for medial and lateral epicondylitis, with one serving as a control. It is rare to have both medial and lateral epicondylitis in the same elbow, so if they have pain with *both* resisted flexion and extension, the test is not diagnostic.

▶ Medical Treatment

Despite the controversy about whether epicondylitis is or is not an inflammatory condition, success can be achieved using NSAIDs in some cases. Stretching can help cure epicondylitis as well. Realize that this condition never occurs in patients younger than 20. It has been hypothesized that this is because the tendon attachments in younger patients are more elastic. Studies have shown that the percentage of elastin in human connective tissue decreases with age. This leads to a loss of elasticity in tendons as they age, making it easier for them to tear. Microscopic tearing of tendon connective tissue is often seen in tissue tendon biopsy samples from patients with epicondylitis, so one theory is that the age-related loss of elasticity leads to microscopic tearing. The goal of stretching for epicondylitis is to try to restore flexibility to the tendon. As you would predict, the stretch for lateral epicondylitis aims to lengthen the extensors, which is done by having the patient straighten their fingers, wrist, and elbow, then, using their other hand, flex the fingers and wrist (Figure 4-28). It is important that the elbow be kept straight because bending the elbow puts slack in the extensors. The opposite stretch is used for medial epicondylitis.

A tennis elbow strap, or band, can also help (Figure 4-29). It works like a capo on the neck of a guitar (see sidebar). Despite

THE "FOREARM CAPO"

A capo is a device used by guitarists to effectively shorten the neck of the guitar (Figure 4-K). It clamps the strings against

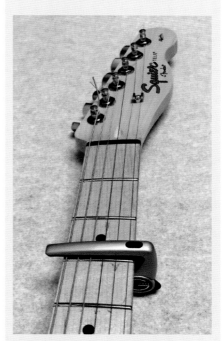

Figure 4-K. A guitar capo. The forearm strap used to treat medial and lateral epicondylitis works in a similar way to reduce the forces at the origins of the common flexor and extensor muscle groups onto the epicondyles of the elbow.

(continued on following page)

the neck, stopping string vibration at that point. The forearm strap used in the treatment of medial and lateral epicondylitis (and the chopat strap used in the treatment of knee patellar tendonitis) keeps the motion and vibration of the muscles beneath it from reaching their bony attachments and causing pain there.

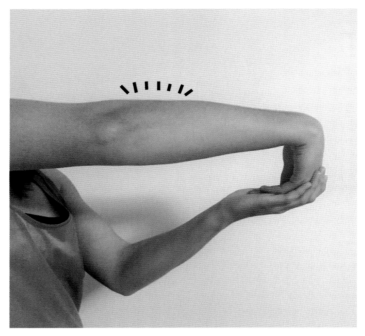

Figure 4-28. The stretch for lateral epicondylitis. With the elbow extended straight, flex the fingers and wrist to stretch the common extensor muscles. The stretch for medial epicondylitis is the opposite: palm up, extend the wrist and outstretched fingers.

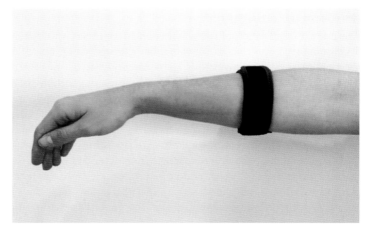

Figure 4-29. A forearm strap can help with the symptoms of medial or lateral epicondylitis by decreasing the tension of the flexor and extensor muscles at their origin on the epicondyles of the elbow. (See sidebar, page 137.)

the fact that it is called a *tennis elbow* strap, it can work for medial epicondylitis (golfer's elbow), too. A rigid, Velcro wrist brace like the one shown in Figure 4-5 can rest wrist flexor/extensor muscles and lessen symptoms as well.

A cortisone shot can be very effective for epicondylitis (learn the simple technique in Chapter 9). Be warned, however: Cortisone injections for medial and lateral epicondylitis have the highest rates of postinjection complications of any of the in-office injection techniques. Injection site pain is the most common complication. It usually sets in 12-24 hours after the injection and can last 24-48 hours. It is not dangerous, and usually responds to ice, NSAIDs, and, in severe cases, narcotics. Local skin changes can occur as well. These include loss of pigmentation, atrophy of the surrounding fat (which makes the epicondyle appear more prominent), and proliferation of fragile cutaneous venous networks that may bleed spontaneously or with minimal trauma. Though they may take months to resolve, these skin changes are temporary, and, in some cases, do not appear until months after the injection. Also, remember that, in the case of injections for medial epicondylitis that contain lidocaine, a 2- to 4-hour period of numbness in the ulnar nerve distribution (small and ring fingers) may occur given the proximity of the medial epicondyle to the ulnar nerve. Though many authors advocate the use of cortisone injections for this condition, a recent study suggested patients who have had an injection for this condition have WORSE outcomes at 1 year despite some short-term improvement.

The treatment of epicondylitis is often frustrating for the patient and the provider. The condition is common and can be very uncomfortable, even debilitating for some patients. To make matters worse, none of the previously mentioned treatments have proven particularly successful. For this reason, there are a host of less orthodox remedies for this condition. Procedures like extracorporeal shock-wave treatment, platelet-rich plasma (PRP) injections, stem cell injections, infrared light treatment, topical laser treatment, application of magnets or copper, and use of a compression sleeve are some examples. None of these treatment options has been proven consistently effective in multiple prospective, randomized, double-blinded clinical trials. As a result, these treatments are not typically covered by standard medical insurance. Many of them are interesting and have compelling anecdotal evidence to back them up and perhaps, with time and more study, will prove to be useful tools in the care of this difficult-to-treat condition.

▶ Surgical Treatment

Like the nonoperative treatments for medial and lateral epicondylitis, surgical treatment has a relatively high failure rate. Many different operations exist, perhaps because no single operation has proven to be particularly successful. A common surgical solution is to partially divide the extensor tendon. A simple 1-cm incision is made in the middle of the tendon perpendicular to its fibers

(Figure 4-30). This small "gap" in the sheet-like tendon has the effect of making it more flexible, like a buttonhole in a shirt (Figure 4-31).

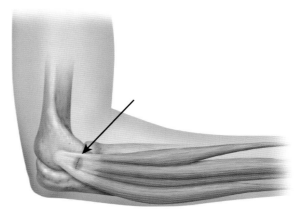

Figure 4-30. Tennis elbow surgery: creating a 1-cm fenestration in the common extensor origin.

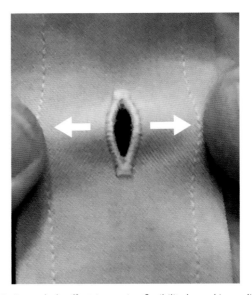

Figure 4-31. Buttonhole effect: increasing flexibility by making a slit.

Olecranon Bursitis

There are several locations in the human body where the skin has to move smoothly and through a large excursion over a bony prominence. The tip of the elbow is one such location (so is the kneecap). In these areas, nature has devised an ingenious bearing system called a *bursa*. Imagine a thin-walled, flexible plastic sack about the size of a plum. The sack is empty and collapsed down upon itself, with only a few drops of slippery, slimy synovial fluid inside it. The bursa sack is interposed between the bony "point" of the elbow (the olecranon process) and the skin. As the skin moves back and forth over the olecranon process with elbow flexion and extension, the two surfaces of the collapsed sack slide and glide on each other with the few drops of synovial fluid between them as a lubricant. Typically, this is a very efficient bearing. In the condition known as olecranon bursitis, the collapsed bursa sack inflates with fluid, creating a prominent, fluctuant, egg-shaped mass (Figure 4-32). If there is a history of trauma, the fluid may be

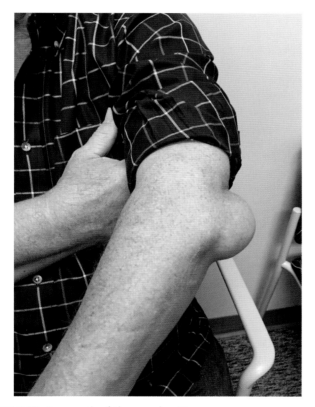

Figure 4-32. An example of olecranon bursitis.

blood. There isn't much soft tissue padding over the olecranon process, so even a mild contusion can rupture a small blood vessel and cause the bursa sack to fill with blood. This condition is called a *hemorrhagic olecranon bursitis,* and it typically resolves with time.

In a few cases of hemorrhagic olecranon bursitis, some of the blood hardens into a pellet of firm, dense scar tissue inside of the bursa sack. This piece of scar tissue mechanically irritates the surfaces of the bursa sack as they slide over each other during normal elbow function. The irritation stimulates the synovial cells in the wall of the bursa to secrete additional synovial fluid, filling the bursa and creating an *inflammatory olecranon bursitis*. An inflammatory olecranon bursitis can be a chronic problem. It may come and go based on activity, or it may stay permanently inflated. If the olecranon bursa becomes infected, either through hematogenous spread or as a result of a foreign object that penetrates the skin and inoculates the inside of the bursa, the result is called a *septic olecranon bursitis*.

Heat, immobilization, and splinting for 1-2 weeks can help resolve hemorrhagic or inflammatory olecranon bursitis. If the bursitis persists or returns, it can be aspirated. An 18-gauge needle is recommended since the fluid is often too thick to pass through a smaller bore needle. Aspirating an olecranon bursa is easy because the target is so close to the skin. Resist the temptation to insert the needle directly into part of the bursa that is directly beneath the skin. This can create a tract that will continuously drain. Instead, choose an insertion point about 2 cm away from the bursa. Push the needle through this 2-cm section of normal, healthy skin and then into the bursa. It is much harder for the bursa fluid to continue to drain through a 2-cm tunnel once the needle has been removed. Avoid inserting the needle on the medial side of the elbow, as this is where the ulnar nerve resides.

Severe pain, redness, and warmth may indicate that the bursa is infected. I recommend aspirating infected olecranon bursas, even if it requires passing the needle through an area of cellulitis. If the fluid you obtain is blood or clear, yellow, benign-appearing inflammatory fluid, it is unlikely that the bursa is infected. If the bursa is not infected, aspirating the fluid may help the condition resolve. Some advocate injecting 20-40 mg of corticosteroid if it is clear that the bursa is not infected.

If the fluid appears purulent or there is any question of a possible infection, do not inject the corticosteroid. Send the aspirate for Gram stain and culture. Rarely, an infected olecranon bursitis can be treated with aspiration and antibiotics. It is more likely, however, that the patient will require surgical excision of the infected olecranon bursa. The olecranon bursa can also be excised in patients who have recurrent hemorrhagic or inflammatory bursitis. Cool fact: Within 6-12 weeks after the bursa is surgically excised, the patient will grow a new, healthy bursa to take its place!

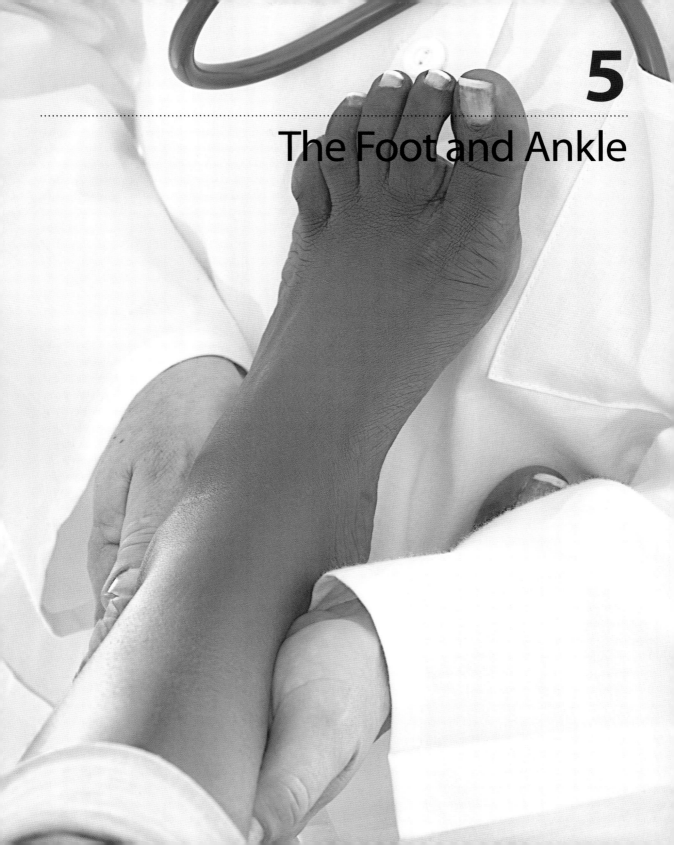

5

The Foot and Ankle

WANT TO SEE MY TIBIALIS ANTERIOR?

Whether you have any medical training or not, chances are good that you can correctly identify a patient's Achilles tendon. But, what about the tibialis anterior, peroneal, and tibialis posterior tendons? The easiest of these is the tibialis anterior (Figure 5-A), which crosses the anterior

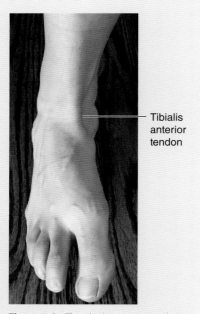

Tibialis anterior tendon

Figure 5-A. The tibialis anterior tendon.

ankle and stands out dramatically as a rope-like band when the ankle is dorsiflexed (extended). The tibialis posterior, which inverts (supinates) the foot, is harder to spot. It is just posterior to the medial malleolus of the ankle and can sometimes be seen or palpated on thin patients as they actively invert their foot. The peroneal tendons (longus and brevis) trace a parallel path posterior to the lateral malleolus and are the hardest to detect on physical exam. If you palpate

(continued on following page)

To start our review of common foot and ankle problems, we begin with some basic anatomy. There are many bones in the foot, and there is no need to memorize the names of all of them, but it is helpful to know the names of the *groups* of bones (Figures 5-1 to 5-6). From distal to proximal, we start with the phalanges, the bones in our toes. Each toe has a distal, a middle, and a proximal phalanx, except the big toe, which only has a distal and a proximal phalanx. Just proximal to the phalanges is the second group of foot bones, the long, slender metatarsal bones. The metatarsals and phalanges account for what is often referred to as the forefoot. Just proximal to the metatarsal bones are a group of small, short bones called the tarsal bones, which make up the midfoot. The hindfoot bones are the talus and the calcaneus, and the talus is the bone that is the "ball" of the ball-and-socket of the ankle. The "socket" of the ankle joint is actually two separate bones. The tibia contributes the roof and the medial sidewall of the socket, and the distal tip of the fibula accounts for the lateral sidewall. At the sidewalls of the ankle joint, the tibia and fibula become a bit thicker and a bit more prominent, creating the hard, bony features of the ankle that we call the medial and lateral malleoli. That's a grand total of 28 bones in the foot and ankle (not including the two tiny sesamoid bones under the big toe!). It seems intuitive that our hands would have a disproportionately high number of bones in them, given the large array of complex motions they have evolved to perform,

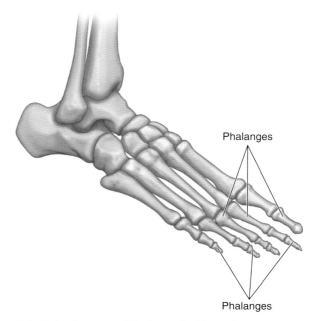

Phalanges

Phalanges

Figure 5-1. Skeletal anatomy of the foot and ankle: phalanges.

the skin just posterior and proximal to the lateral malleolus on a thin patient who is everting (also called pronating) their foot, you may feel the peroneus longus tendon.

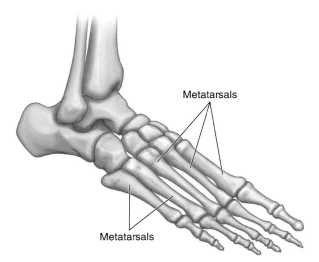

Figure 5-2. Skeletal anatomy of the foot and ankle: metatarsals.

but why the skeletal structure of our feet is so complex is harder to understand.

Despite this apparent overabundance of bones, there aren't any muscles in the foot and ankle that are important enough to deserve mention in an anatomic review as basic as this one. In simplest terms, the foot and ankle only move in four directions: flexion (up), extension (down), inversion (toward the midline,

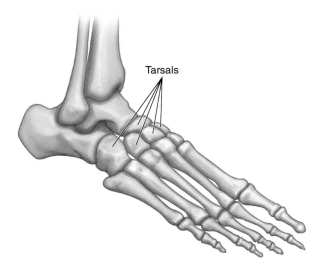

Figure 5-3. Skeletal anatomy of the foot and ankle: tarsals.

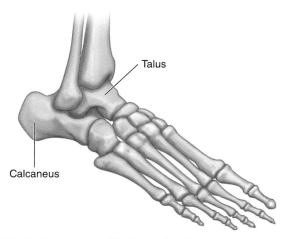

Figure 5-4. Skeletal anatomy of the foot and ankle: calcaneus, talus.

sometimes called supination), and eversion (away from the midline, sometimes called pronation). For the most part, these four motions result from forces applied to the foot and ankle by the calf muscles via their specific tendons. For example, the downward

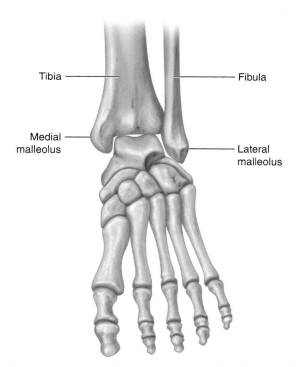

Figure 5-5. Skeletal anatomy of the foot and ankle: medial and lateral malleolus.

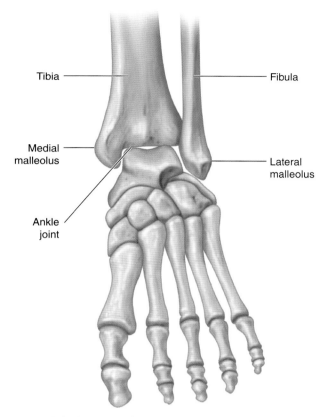

Tibia

Fibula

Medial malleolus

Lateral malleolus

Ankle joint

Figure 5-6. Skeletal anatomy of the foot and ankle: tibia, fibula, ankle joint.

motion of ankle flexion (sometimes referred to as plantar flexion) occurs when the calcaneus is pulled proximally by the Achilles tendon and the gastrocnemius and soleus muscles attached to it. Similarly, ankle upward extension (sometimes referred to as dorsiflexion) results from contraction of the tibialis anterior muscle (see sidebar, page 146), and inversion/supination and eversion/pronation result from contraction of the tibialis posterior and peroneal muscles, respectively.

The only ligaments worth noting in this discussion are the ankle-stabilizing ligaments. The ankle joint moves freely in the flexion-extension plane of motion but does not move much from side to side. This side-to-side motion occurs primarily at the hindfoot joint below the ankle, between the talus and the calcaneus, and is limited at the ankle joint by the ankle-stabilizing ligaments. There are three ligaments on the lateral side of the ankle joint and one on the medial side (Figure 5-7). These ligaments are covered in more detail in the ankle sprain section of this chapter.

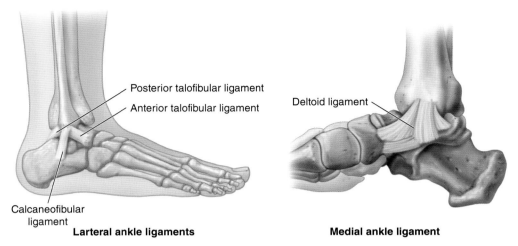

Figure 5-7. The lateral and medial ligaments of the ankle.

MORTON'S NEUROMA

Figure 5-8 shows how the medial and lateral plantar nerves branch into the common digital nerves, which then branch into the proper digital nerves to provide sensory innervation to the medial and lateral sides of the toes. On the distal end of each metatarsal bone, there is a bulbous mass of bone known as the metatarsal head. The common digital nerves pass between the metatarsal heads as they bifurcate into their terminal branches: the proper digital nerves.

WHY THE THIRD WEBSPACE?

Morton's neuroma can occur at any of the webspaces of the foot, but the third webspace is by far the most common. The anatomy of the foot may explain why.

As we walk, the metatarsal bones in our feet move up and down like the keys on a piano. Metatarsals 1, 2, and 3 are each jointed to their own tarsal (cuneiform) bone, whereas metatarsals 4 and 5 are both jointed to the same tarsal (cuboid) bone. This is illustrated by the blue shade in Figure 5-B. The result is that metatarsals 4 and 5 are more rigidly bound together, creating less motion between themselves and relatively more motion between metatarsal number 4 and its more mobile neighbor, metatarsal number 3. It is thought that the increased motion between the bulbous heads on the ends of metatarsals 3 and 4 is responsible for the higher propensity for nerve

(continued on following page)

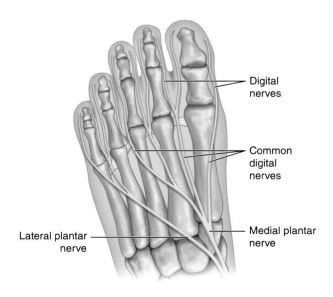

Figure 5-8. The plantar sensory nerves of the foot.

As we walk, there is movement between adjacent metatarsal heads, and that movement can create the inflammatory changes that result in a Morton's neuroma. While this can occur between any two adjacent metatarsal heads, it is most common in the webspace between the third and fourth toes, where the nerve is sandwiched between the third and fourth metatarsal heads (see sidebar, page 150). Figure 5-9 shows an inflamed, swollen

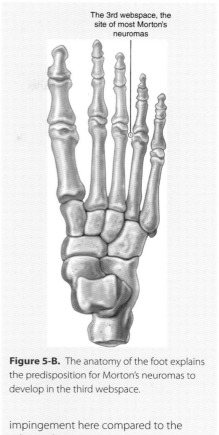

The 3rd webspace, the site of most Morton's neuromas

Figure 5-B. The anatomy of the foot explains the predisposition for Morton's neuromas to develop in the third webspace.

impingement here compared to the other webspaces.

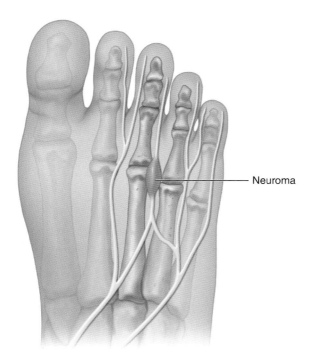

Neuroma

Figure 5-9. The classic location for a Morton's neuroma.

Morton's neuroma in the third webspace. Patients with a Morton's neuroma usually complain of pain that "feels like a pebble" on the bottom of their foot. The pain may radiate into the toes distal to that webspace, and symptoms are usually worse in high-heeled shoes or shoes with a narrow toe box. The nerve may malfunction, causing numbness or tingling.

▶ Physical Exam

The mass may be large enough to splay the toes (Figure 5-10). You may detect a loss of sensation to light touch, and some of the bigger masses can be palpated on physical exam. If you hold the metatarsal heads of two adjacent toes and move them in opposite directions, up and down several times, you can often re-create the patient's pain. This is called the *metatarsal shift test*.

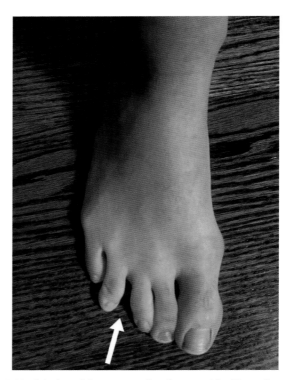

Figure 5-10. Splaying of the toes occasionally seen with a Morton's neuroma.

▶ *Imaging Studies*

X-rays aren't likely to show anything, other than, perhaps, a widening of the space between the metatarsal heads. A magnetic resonance image (MRI) may show inflammatory changes in and around the neuroma.

▶ *Medical Treatment*

Shoes that subject the metatarsal heads to high stress can precipitate impingement of the nerve and result in a Morton's neuroma (Figure 5-11). High-heeled shoes are known for loading the metatarsal heads, and the toe box on these shoes is typically narrow, crowding the metatarsal heads against one another. Narrow, high-heeled shoes create the perfect environment for the development of this condition. Changing to a wide shoe with a low heel can make a big difference, as can adding a metatarsal support (Figure 5-12). Metatarsal supports can be applied to the skin of the foot, as in Figure 5-12, or built into the shoe. These supports transfer weight-bearing forces off the metatarsal heads and into the arch. A cortisone injection into the space between the metatarsal heads can decrease inflammation and help the symptoms of a Morton's neuroma resolve. (See Chapter 9 for the injection technique for Morton's neuroma.)

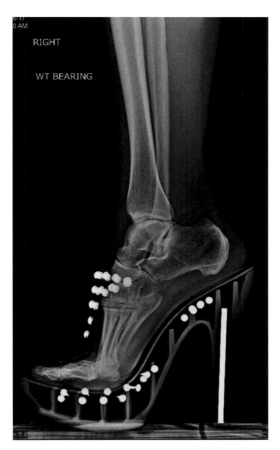

Figure 5-11. High-heeled shoes expose the metatarsal heads to high compressive forces.

▶ *Surgical Treatment*

The surgical treatment of Morton's neuroma involves making a small incision over the involved webspace on the dorsum of the foot, exposing the neuroma, and then resecting it (Figure 5-13). The entire neuroma is removed by cutting the proximal common digital nerve and both of the distal digital nerve branches. Numbness on one side of each toe results, but most patients prefer this to the pain of the neuroma. No motor deficit results because this is a purely sensory nerve.

PLANTAR FASCIITIS

Running along the plantar surface of our feet is a tough, stiff band of dense connective tissue called the *plantar fascia* (Figure 5-14). It originates from the plantar surface of the calcaneus and inserts onto the plantar surfaces of the metatarsal heads. Like the string on a bow, it spans the space between the hindfoot and forefoot, and

SAGGING AT NIGHT

Plantar grade is the term we use to describe the position of our foot when we stand (Figure 5-C). The sole of the

(continued on following page)

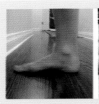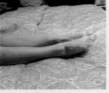

Figure 5-C. The position of the foot when standing (left) and sleeping (right).

foot and the leg form an angle of about 90 degrees. At 90 degrees, the Achilles tendon and plantar fascia are both somewhat stretched. When we sleep, our foot naturally drifts into a position with the toes pointed downward, relaxing the Achilles tendon and plantar fascia. After a night of sleeping with our feet in this position, the Achilles and plantar fascia are shorter than when they are stretched out. When we take our first step, these structures are abruptly stretched. If they are inflamed and lack flexibility and compliance, the abrupt stretch that accompanies the first step out of bed in the morning can be quite painful. This is why patients with Achilles tendonitis and plantar fasciitis often complain of pain that is worse with the first few steps of the day. A night splint (see Figure 5-18B) can help by maintaining a gentle stretch across the plantar fascia and Achilles tendon during the night, so that the first steps don't strain them as severely. A morning stretch routine may help as well. Something as simple as looping a towel over the ball of the foot and pulling the ball of the foot toward one's chest to stretch the foot and ankle for 30 seconds to a minute can help in the treatment of plantar fasciitis and Achilles tendonitis.

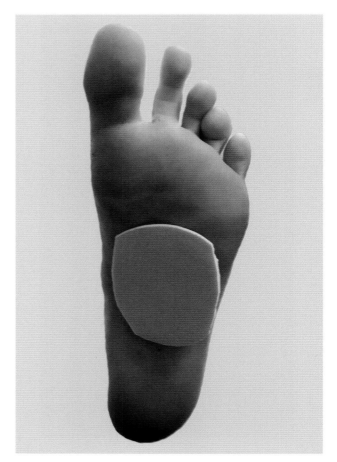

Figure 5-12. A metatarsal pad with an adhesive backing that allows it to stick to the surface of the foot. The metatarsal pad transfers the weight-bearing forces off the metatarsal heads and onto the arch of the foot.

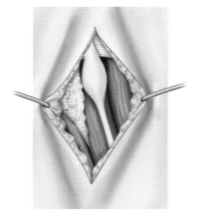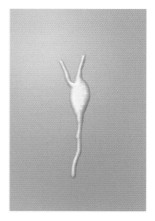

Figure 5-13. Surgical removal of a Morton's neuroma.

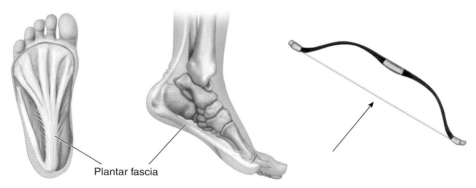

Figure 5-14. The plantar fascia, which spans the bottom of the foot, is a tense band of connective tissue that acts like the string on a bow to help maintain the arch.

it helps maintain the arch of the sole of the foot. In the condition known as plantar fasciitis, the plantar fascia becomes inflamed, usually at its attachment to the calcaneus, and this creates pain that can be quite intense. The condition usually affects patients who are over the age of 40, and men are more likely to be affected than women. The classic symptom is one of heel pain that is worse on first putting weight on the heel in the morning (see sidebar, pages 153-154).

▶ *Physical Exam*

On physical examination, the patient's foot with plantar fasciitis is usually tender to palpation on the plantar surface of the foot, where the plantar fascia attaches to the calcaneus (see arrow in Figure 5-15). The plantar fascia may also feel tight to palpation as well.

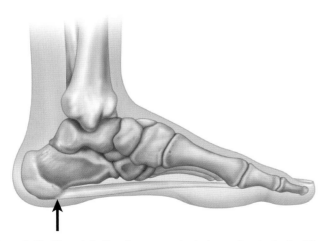

Figure 5-15. The point of tenderness on physical exam for plantar fasciitis.

THE MYTH OF THE BONE SPUR

One of the changes that can be seen in inflamed tissue is ischemia. These ischemic changes can result in a localized drop in pH, which can cause serum calcium and phosphate to precipitate and form calcific deposits in soft tissue. In the case of plantar fasciitis, the chronic inflammatory changes occur at the insertion point of the plantar fascia onto the calcaneus, and the fascia at this point may calcify, forming the plantar heel spur (see Figure 5-16). It is important to note that the plantar heel spur is the *result* of the chronic, local ischemic conditions associated with plantar fasciitis, not the *cause* of them.

▶ Imaging

On a lateral x-ray of the foot, you may see a small, calcified protuberance where the plantar fascia attaches to the calcaneus (Figure 5-16). This finding is known as the plantar heel spur.

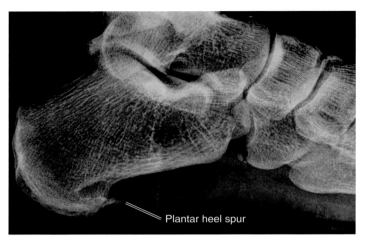

Plantar heel spur

Figure 5-16. A lateral x-ray of the foot showing a plantar heel spur (*Licensed from Shutterstock*).

Because it appears sharp and it is located in exactly the place of maximal pain in plantar fasciitis, it is often assumed that the plantar spur is the cause of the heel pain in plantar fasciitis. This is not true (see sidebar).

▶ Medical Treatment

Because inflammation appears to be the cause of plantar fasciitis in some patients, treatment with nonsteroidal anti-inflammatory drugs (NSAIDs) does work for certain individuals, especially those who present soon after initially experiencing symptoms. A standard "first-line" treatment would include NSAIDs combined with stretches designed to stretch the plantar fascia and Achilles Tendon. Standing with the ball of the foot on a stair riser and letting the heel drop down is a simple and inexpensive way to accomplish this stretch (Figure 5-17). Heel pad inserts can also help. Some advocate massage techniques that aim to increase the flexibility of the plantar fascia. Night splints can play a role (see sidebar), and, in extreme cases, a short leg walking cast can be used to rigidly immobilize the foot and ankle in a 90-degree, plantar-grade position (Figure 5-18). This keeps the plantar fascia on tension. Wearing cowboy boots, or other boots with a modest heel, will raise the heel and allow the Achilles and plantar fascia to relax (essentially the opposite effect of the stairstep/heel drop stretch). While this foot position may afford some relief of the symptoms associated

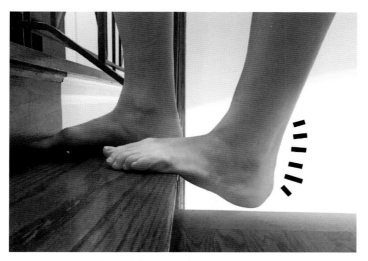

Figure 5-17. A good stretch for plantar fasciitis and Achilles tendonitis. Let the heel drop down and hold it for 30 seconds to a minute 10 times a day.

with applying tension to the plantar fascia, it does not promote flexibility or increase the compliance of the plantar fascia and, as such, may be a poor long-term solution. A cortisone injection tends to work well, but it is one of the most painful injections in all of orthopedics, and it is technically more difficult to administer than cortisone injections in other locations. Care must be taken not to inject the plantar fat pad just deep to the skin on the plantar surface of the foot. Injected corticosteroids can cause this important fatty cushion to atrophy, making walking more difficult and painful. For more details on the technique for injecting the plantar fascia, see Chapter 9.

▶ *Surgical Treatment*

The surgical treatment of plantar fasciitis is relatively straightforward and simple (Figure 5-19). An incision is made on the medial or lateral side of the heel (incisions on the plantar surface of the foot are to be avoided, as they can leave a firm, rigid scar on the weight-bearing part of the foot). The plantar fascia is identified at its attachment to the calcaneus, and divided. There are two schools of thought regarding whether it is best to fully or partially divide the plantar fascia. If the plantar fascia is completely divided, the results are better for pain relief, but there are concerns that complete division of the plantar fascia may result in arch collapse over time. Advocates of complete release of the plantar fascia point out that there does not appear to be any ill consequence of the flat foot deformity, and that there are many patients out there with flat foot deformities, acquired and congenital, who are completely asymptomatic. While the incidence

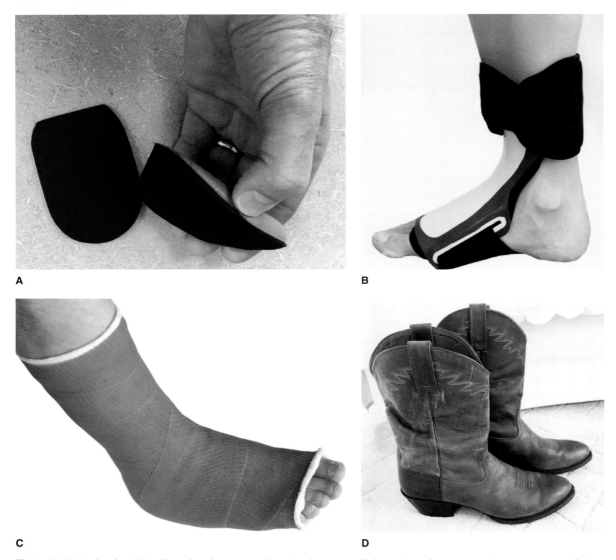

Figure 5-18. Heel pads, night splints, short leg casts, and cowboy boots can all play a role in the nonoperative management of plantar fasciitis (*C: Licensed from Shutterstock*).

of a flat foot deformity acquired in this way is less if the plantar fascia is partially released, the results of the operation, in terms of pain relief, are not as dramatic.

ACHILLES TENDONITIS

Achilles tendonitis and plantar fasciitis are very similar (Figure 5-20). Patient age and gender demographics are similar, and the pathophysiology is similar. In both conditions, an age-related loss of flexibility

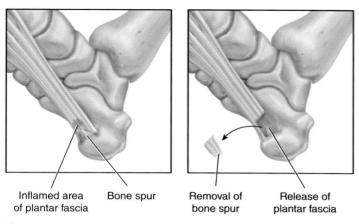

Inflamed area   Bone spur   Removal of   Release of
of plantar fascia   bone spur   plantar fascia

Figure 5-19. Surgical release of the plantar fascia.

in the tissue sets up chronic, post-traumatic inflammatory changes that create pain. The treatment options for Achilles tendonitis are essentially the same, with an emphasis on calf stretches, night splints, NSAIDs, and, occasionally, casting. One important difference is that *cortisone injections are not recommended in or around the Achilles tendon.* Injections here can predispose to Achilles tendon rupture.

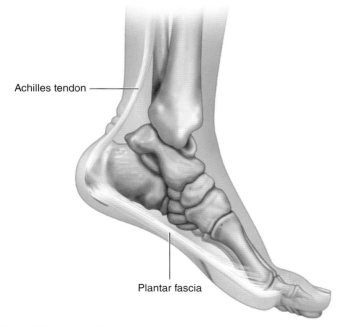

Achilles tendon

Plantar fascia

Figure 5-20. The Achilles tendon and plantar fascia.

Surgical procedures exist for Achilles tendonitis, but they are rarely recommended and are not particularly successful. The most popular procedure is to debride inflammatory tissue from between the load-bearing fibers of the tendon.

HAMMERTOES, BUNIONS, AND CORNS

This group of foot deformities of hammertoes, bunions, and corns is fairly common, especially in older patients. As we age, the joints in our toes are prone to deformities that produce bony prominences that can cause pain and skin ulceration. The bunion deformity occurs when the proximal phalanx of the big toe deviates laterally and the first metatarsal deviates medially (Figure 5-21). This results in a medial bony prominence at the

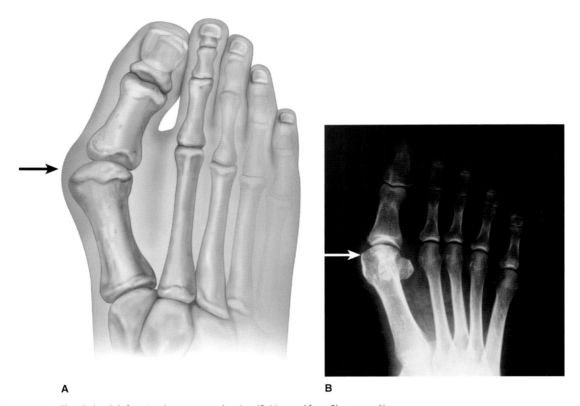

A   **B**

Figure 5-21. The skeletal deformity that creates a bunion (*B: Licensed from Shutterstock*).

metatarsal-phalangeal joint that can rub against the inside of the shoe and cause pain. Hammertoes result from a combination of extension at the metatarsal-phalangeal joint and flexion at one or more of the interphalangeal joints (Figure 5-22). Bunions and hammertoes are typically rigid, inflexible deformities. They create

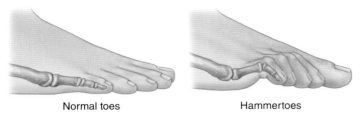

Normal toes   Hammertoes

Figure 5-22. The skeletal deformity that creates a hammertoe.

areas of abnormal contact and abnormal pressure on the skin of the toes and foot against the shoe. The skin can break down in these areas, creating discomfort and an opportunity for infection. Corns and calluses are the skin changes that result from the toes rubbing against the shoe (Figure 5-23). Left untreated, corns and calluses can break down to form skin ulcers.

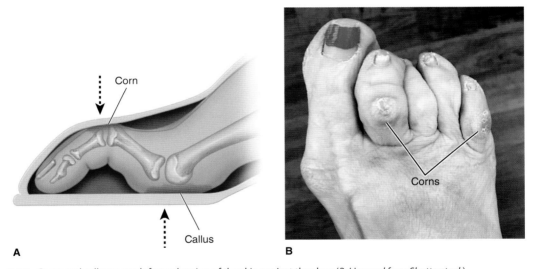

Corn

Callus

A   **B**

Figure 5-23. Corns and calluses result from abrasion of the skin against the shoe (*B: Licensed from Shutterstock*).

▶ *Medical Treatment*

Bunions, corns, and hammertoes are all very common and can be completely asymptomatic. They only need to be treated if there is significant pain or the threat of skin breakdown, both of which can usually be avoided by padding the skin or modifying the shoe. Bunion and corn pads are appliances that shield the skin from rubbing against the inside of the shoe (Figure 5-24). Orthopedic shoes have a wide, roomy toe box to allow room for bony deformities like bunions and hammertoes (see adjacent Figure). They are probably the least attractive shoes ever manufactured, but they keep the skin from rubbing against the shoe and breaking down.

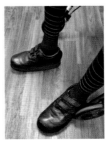

Figure. Orthopedic shoes: soft, wide roomy toe, and really ugly.

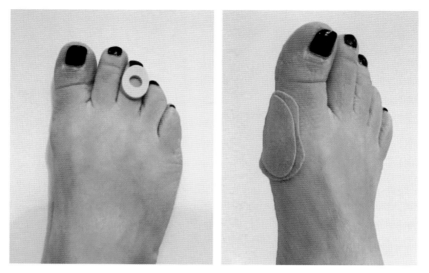

Figure 5-24. Adhesive-backed corn pads (left) and medial bunion pads (right) can prevent pain and skin breakdown.

▶ *Surgical Treatment*

If nonoperative treatment is unsuccessful in preventing pain and skin ulceration, there are surgical solutions that aim to correct the deformities caused by bunions and hammertoes. These operations usually involve cutting the bones of the foot in one or more places, straightening angular deformities, and holding the bones in the corrected position with plates, wires, or screws (Figure 5-25).

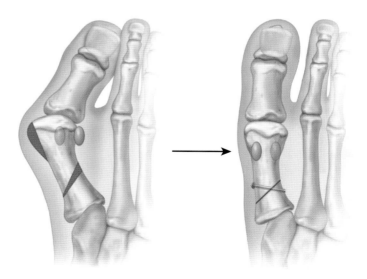

Figure 5-25. An example of the surgical correction of a bunion. Several different procedures exist.

POSTERIOR TIBIAL TENDON DYSFUNCTION (adult-acquired flatfoot deformity)

A common source of medial arch pain and acquired flatfoot deformity in adults is posterior tibial tendon dysfunction (PTTD) (Figure 5-26). This is a progressive, degenerative condition that

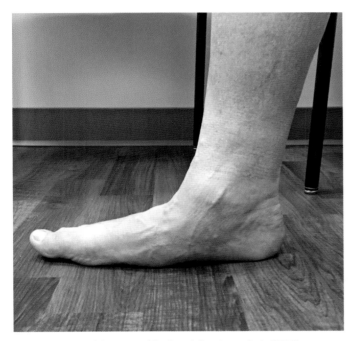

Figure 5-26. The adult-acquired flatfoot deformity typical of PTTD.

affects the tibialis posterior tendon, a major tendon that starts in the lower part of the medial leg and runs inferior to the medial malleolus to insert into the bones of the medial arch of the foot (Figure 5-27). The tibialis posterior tendon and the muscle from which it originates (the tibialis posterior muscle in the upper medial calf) play an important role in stabilizing the hindfoot and maintaining the arch. In PTTD, the tendon becomes thick, swollen, tender, and inflamed. As the disease progresses, the swollen tendon becomes too big for its sheath, and it can no longer glide freely in its sheath, eliminating it as a dynamic stabilizer of the arch and hindfoot. Without a functional tibialis posterior muscle and tendon, the arch collapses, and the heel begins to tilt laterally toward the fibula. Initially, the collapsed arch is still flexible enough that if you put an arch support in the shoe, the foot will conform to the arch support, and the arch will be restored. Left

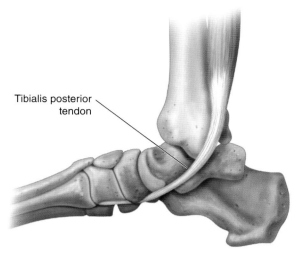

Figure 5-27. The anatomy of the tibialis posterior muscle and tendon.

untreated, the collapsed arch deformity becomes rigid and is not correctable without surgery. The dysfunctional tendon may fray, partially tear, or even completely rupture.

▶ *Physical Exam*

If you are seeing a patient 50 years of age or older with atraumatic medial arch pain, PTTD is the most likely diagnosis. To confirm the diagnosis on physical exam, examine the patient in shorts, standing with shoes and socks removed. Look at the patient's heels from behind (Figure 5-28). If the arch has collapsed due to PTTD,

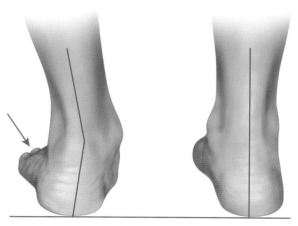

Figure 5-28. The PTTD deformity involves lateral tilting of the heel and a "too many toes" sign from external rotation of the foot. It is best seen by examining the standing patient from behind, where it appears that too many toes are visable on the lateral side of the foot.

you will notice that the heel is tilted laterally, and the foot is rotated externally, creating the "too many toes" sign. External rotation of the foot allows you to see more of the lateral toes than you see on the unaffected foot. Another helpful test is to ask the patient to stand on one foot and then rise up onto the ball of the foot, raising the heel up off of the floor. This is easy to do on a normal foot but nearly impossible for a foot with PTTD.

▶ Medical Treatment

If diagnosed early enough, a simple, molded arch support or University of California Berkley Laboratories (UCBL) hindfoot brace can effectively substitute for the dysfunctional tibialis posterior muscle and tendon. These appliances can restore functional support to the arch and hindfoot and minimize gait abnormalities and pain. There may also be a role for resisted inversion exercises that aim to strengthen the tibialis posterior (Figure 5-29). As the

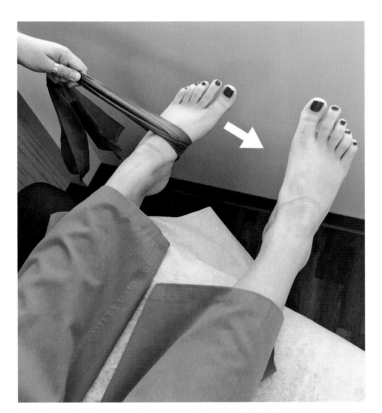

Figure 5-29. Using an elastic band to strengthen the tibialis posterior muscle.

disease progresses and the deformity becomes more rigid, surgery may be necessary to restore the arch, hindfoot stability, and normal gait pattern.

ANKLE INJURIES: SPRAINS AND FRACTURES

Ankle sprains and fractures both result from deforming forces applied across the ankle joint. In the case of an ankle sprain, these forces tear the connective tissue bands (ligaments) that stabilize the ankle joint (Figures 5-30 to 5-32). The most common

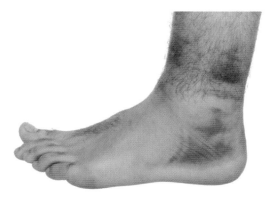

Figure 5-30. A typical ankle injury: Is it a sprain or a fracture? (*Licensed from Shutterstock*).

deforming force is an inversion (supination) injury, in which the sole of the foot is forcibly turned medially, toward the midline. This position of the ankle can tear the lateral ankle ligaments. The ligament that is torn most often when the ankle is sprained is

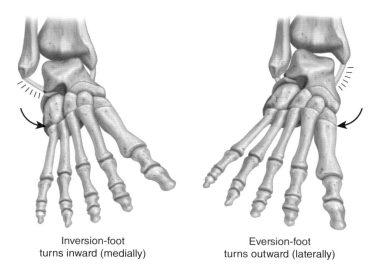

Inversion-foot
turns inward (medially)

Eversion-foot
turns outward (laterally)

Figure 5-31. The ankle ligaments that are torn in inversion and eversion injuries.

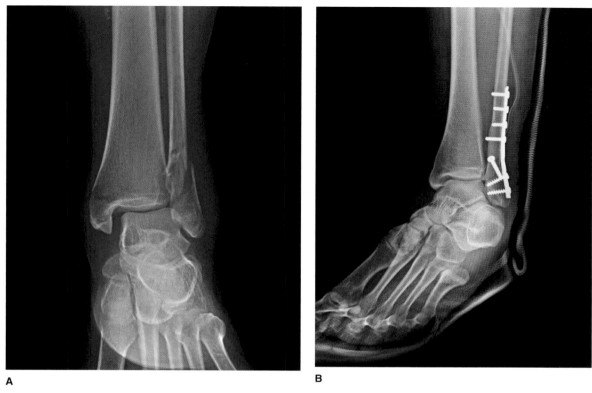

A   **B**

Figure 5-36. A displaced fracture of the lateral malleolus (**A**) and the result of an open reduction, internal fixation procedure to treat it (**B**) (*Licensed from Shutterstock*).

after an open reduction, internal fixation procedure. The goal of ankle fracture treatment is to ensure that the fracture heals in an anatomic position without significant displacement. This requires that we recognize which injuries are sprains and which are fractures. That is easy to do with an x-ray, but it is not practical or cost-effective to x-ray every ankle injury we encounter. The Ottawa rules are a set of guidelines that can help us determine which ankle injuries require an x-ray (Figure 5-37). The rules only apply to patients with malleolar ankle pain. If the patient is over 55 years old, x-rays are indicated because patients in this age group have softer bone that can fracture without much trauma. Low-energy fractures have less impressive clinical findings and are more likely to be mistaken for sprains. The designers of the Ottawa rules also observed that the inability to bear weight correlates with the presence of a fracture. According to the guidelines, patients with pain at any point along the posterior half of the medial or lateral malleolus should be x-rayed. Remember that most sprains involve the ATFL, which is an anterior structure. Patients with ATFL sprains will have tenderness over the anterior half of the lateral malleolus,

"THE CLASSICS": COMMON CAUSES OF COMMON INJURIES

Tennis ➔ Achilles tendon rupture
Bicycle crash ➔ Clavicle fracture
Water skiing ➔ Hamstring tear

THOMPSON'S TEST

Thompson's test for Achilles tendon ruptures takes advantage of the fact that the posterior calf muscles are shaped like a cone, with the point of the cone pointing inferiorly (Figure 5-E). If you squeeze

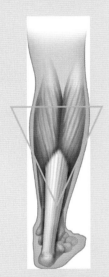

Figure 5-E. The triangle-shaped muscles of the posterior calf.

the calf on a normal, uninjured patient (try this!), the slippery, cone-shaped calf muscles slide out of your hand and move proximally, toward the knee. As the muscles glide proximally, they tug on the Achilles tendon and pull the heel proximally, which plantar flexes the foot. If the

(continued on following page)

The Ottawa rules

• History of trauma and malleolar ankle pain

and any *one* of:

• Age greater than 55
• Inability to bear weight
• Tender over posterior 6 cm of medial *or* lateral malleolus

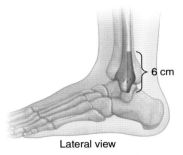

Lateral view

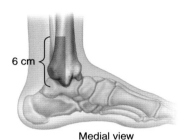

6 cm

Medial view

Figure 5-37. The Ottawa rules regarding which ankle injuries should be screened with an x-ray to look for fractures.

but not the posterior half. Patients with a lateral malleolus fracture will have tenderness at all points anteriorly and posteriorly along the lateral malleolus. In addition to the Ottawa ankle rules, I recommend taking x-rays of ankle injuries that occur in patients with sensory deficits, such as diabetic neuropathy, that make it difficult for them to accurately perceive pain in their extremities.

There are two foot and ankle injuries that can be mistaken for ankle sprains and, if missed, result in poor outcomes. The first is an Achilles tendon rupture (see sidebar). The second is a proximal fifth metatarsal fracture, also called a "Jones fracture." If your patient with an "ankle sprain" doesn't have malleolar ankle pain, they may have one of these two conditions. Patients who sustain an Achilles tendon rupture typically report a violent "pop" in the posterior calf or heel at the time of injury. They usually have tenderness along the Achilles tendon, and, in some cases, a defect in the tendon can be palpated. A clever physical exam test used to diagnose an Achilles tendon rupture is the *Thompson's test* (see sidebar). Achilles tendon ruptures are usually repaired surgically, and the results of that operation are compromised if more than a week or two passes between the time of injury and the time of surgery. For this reason, it is best not to miss an Achilles tendon rupture.

Fifth metatarsal fractures, or Jones fractures, are also often mistaken for ankle sprains. They actually aren't ankle injuries at all, but they commonly result from the same types of twisting injuries that cause ankle sprains. Patients with these fractures will have tenderness over the lateral border of the midfoot and, on x-ray, have a fracture at the junction of the shaft and the proximal neck of the fifth metatarsal (Figure 5-38). The lateral border

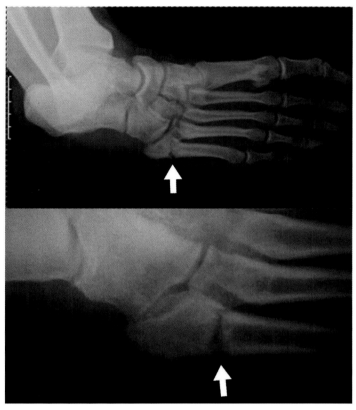

Figure 5-38. An x-ray of the foot demonstrating a Jones fracture of the fifth metatarsal.

of the foot bears a great deal of our weight when we walk (think of the footprint you leave when you walk barefoot in the sand), and this particular fracture requires that patients be treated with crutches and be non–weight bearing for 6 weeks. If this fracture is mistaken for a sprain and the patient is allowed to bear weight as tolerated, the bone may not heal, and the patient may develop a painful nonunion at the fracture site. So, if your patient sustains a twisting injury to their foot and they have tenderness over the proximal end of the fifth metatarsal on the lateral border of their foot, it is probably a good idea to order a set of x-rays to screen for a Jones fracture.

Achilles is torn, the muscles are no longer connected to the heel, and no motion is observed (Figure 5-F). This test is impor-

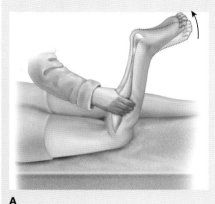

A

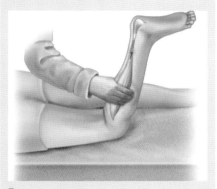

B

Figure 5-F. Thompson's test to detect an Achilles tendon rupture: Place the patient prone and gently squeeze the calf muscles of each leg. Because it is shaped like a cone, or triangle, the muscle will slide proximally when squeezed (imagine squeezing a wet, cone-shaped bar of soap). If the Achilles tendon is intact, the foot will plantar flex when the calf is squeezed (A). If it is torn, the foot won't move (B).

tant because a patient with a complete rupture of the Achilles tendon can still actively plantar flex the foot on command by using their toe flexor muscles and tendons, so their ability to do this does not rule out an Achilles tendon rupture.

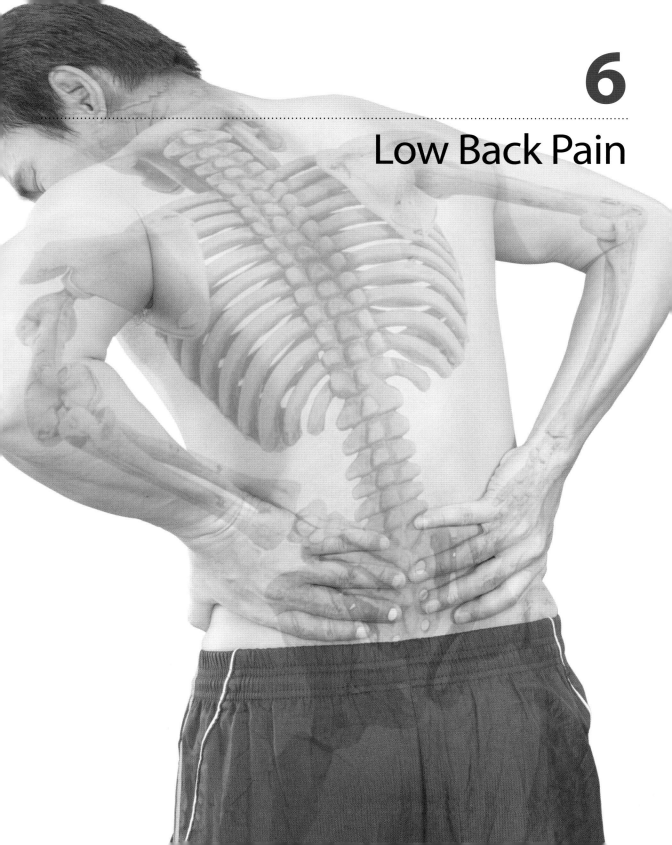

6

Low Back Pain

Despite countless recent advances in diagnosis and treatment, low back pain remains one of the most challenging conditions in all of orthopedics. The results of both surgical and nonsurgical treatments often fall short of patient expectations, making low back pain a frustrating diagnosis for patients and providers alike. The goal of this chapter is to provide a practical, logical, and evidence-based approach to patients with this challenging condition.

ANATOMY

The basic unit in the anatomy of the spine is the vertebra (Figure 6-1). A single vertebra has a solid mass of bone anteriorly called the *vertebral body* and a complicated array of bony spines and prominences posteriorly called the *posterior elements*. In the middle, there is an open passageway called the spinal canal. The spinal canal starts at the foramen magnum, the opening at

THE KILLER CURVE

It has long been observed that two disks in the lumbar spine account for over 90% of back problems: the disk between L4 and L5 and the disk between L5 and S1. If we look at Figure 6-A, we can understand one possible explanation why.

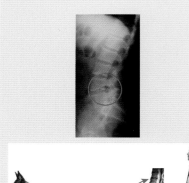

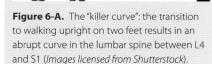

Figure 6-A. The "killer curve": the transition to walking upright on two feet results in an abrupt curve in the lumbar spine between L4 and S1 (*Images licensed from Shutterstock*).

Though it is impossible to prove, there is a theory that the high incidence of back problems at these levels results from the change in loads and forces on the spine that occurred when humans evolved from walking on all fours to standing upright on two feet. This postural change introduced a "kink" in the spinal column between L4 and the sacrum, subjecting the two disks and the facet joints at this level to unusually high stress, increasing the incidence of structural failure here.

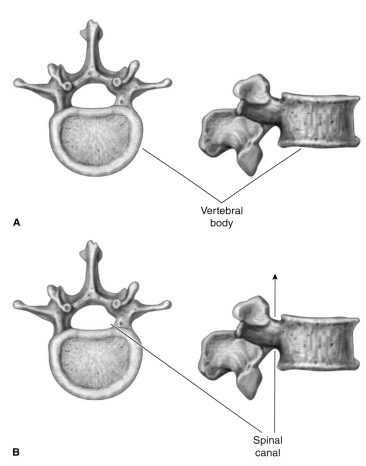

A

B

Vertebral body

Spinal canal

Figure 6-1. Anatomy of a vertebra.

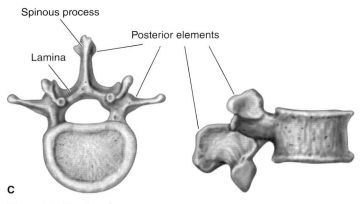

Spinous process

Posterior elements

Lamina

C

Figure 6-1. (*Continued*)

the base of the skull where the brain stops and the spinal cord begins, and it continues all the way down to the coccyx. Adjacent vertebrae are stacked one on top of the other, and together, they form the skeletal structure of our spines: a long sheath of bony "armor" to protect our fragile spinal cord and nerve roots and a structural frame to support our body mass (Figure 6-2). For most

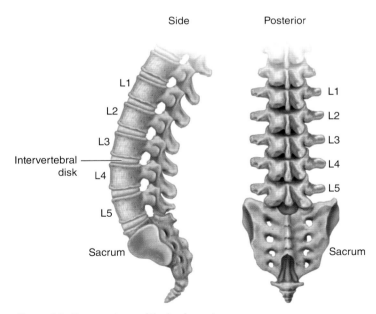

Side   Posterior

L1

L2

L3

Intervertebral
disk   L4

L5

Sacrum

L1

L2

L3

L4

L5

Sacrum

Figure 6-2. Bony anatomy of the lumbar spine.

of the lumbar spine, the spinal canal contains a collection of nerve roots, not the spinal cord. Figure 6-3 shows that the spinal cord ends at approximately the level of the second lumbar vertebra, and

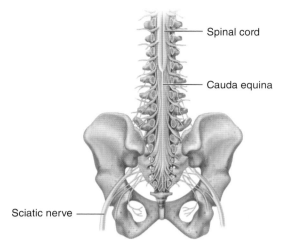

Figure 6-3. The transition from spinal cord to cauda equina in the lumbar spine.

that, below this level, the spinal canal contains a bundle of nerve roots called the cauda equina. Each vertebra is linked to the vertebrae above and below it by firm but flexible connections that allow motion in this otherwise-rigid bony column. In the front, the tissue that connects adjacent vertebrae is called the *intervertebral disk*. Each disk consists of a tough, rubbery peripheral ring known as the *annulus fibrosus* and a soft, jelly-like center known as the *nucleus pulposus* (Figure 6-4). Behind the spinal canal, the

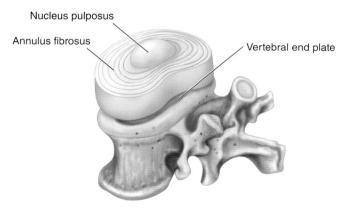

Figure 6-4. Anatomy of an intervertebral disk.

posterior elements of adjacent vertebrae form articulated connections known as the *facet joints*.

This intricate assembly of bones, connective tissue, and neural elements is what we call the *lumbar spine*, and it is depicted in

Figure 6-5. While problems related to the cervical and thoracic spine do account for a percentage of patients' complaints, certainly the vast majority of spine-related problems arise from the lumbar spine, specifically from the lower part of the lumbar spine. It is estimated that over 90% of low back pain comes from pathology at the L4-L5 and L5-S1 levels (see sidebar on page 176 for details).

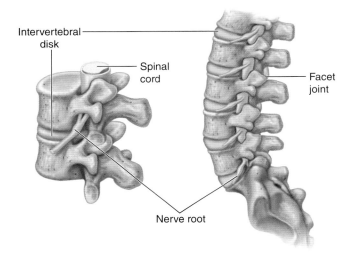

Figure 6-5. Lumbar spine anatomy.

LOW BACK PAIN (WITHOUT RADICULOPATHY)

Low back pain that does not radiate down the lower extremities (below the knees) and is not associated with numbness, tingling, or weakness is relatively common. It may be the result of a muscle strain, facet joint arthritis, or degenerative disk disease.

The intervertebral disks of the spine, especially those between L4 and S1, are continuously exposed to destructive loads and forces as we flex, extend, rotate, compress, and distract our spinal columns with the motions we make on a daily basis. In children, the disks and other supportive structures of the spine are young, strong, and flexible. Low back pain in children is rare, and, when it occurs, it should be investigated thoroughly. Causes of low back pain in children under 10 include infection of an intervertebral disk, leukemia, and scoliosis. Though it is rare in young children, low back pain is quite common in patients over 30. It is said to affect 60%-80% of the adult population at some time in their lives. As we age, the disks and associated supportive structures in our spines wear out and deteriorate. The nucleus pulposus loses much of its water content, and the collagen fibers of the annulus fibrosis begin to fray and fail. These degenerative changes appear to be an inevitable part of the aging process and can be expected to occur at all levels throughout the spine as patients age into their 80s, 90s, and beyond. Magnetic resonance imaging (MRI) studies in patients in these age groups typically show nucleus pulposus dehydration, loss of disk space height, and other signs of disk degeneration. It has been proposed that these degenerative disk changes are the cause of low back pain in some patients, but back pain is certainly present in many patients who lack these degenerative changes, and these degenerative changes are often seen at one or more levels in the spines of patients with little or no back pain.

Alternatively, low back pain may result from a strain of one or more of the many muscles that support the lumbar spine. Figure 6-6 shows the complex assembly of muscles in the low back. Overuse

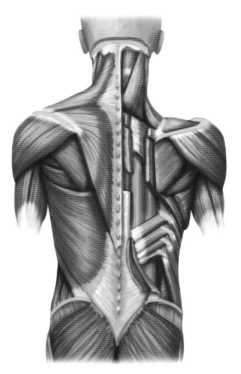

Figure 6-6. The bones of the lumbar spine are supported by a complex system of numerous paraspinal muscles.

of these muscles or poor lifting ergonomics can cause the muscles or their insertions onto the bones and fascia of the spine to become inflamed, resulting in pain and stiffness. Facet joint arthritis may also cause lumbar back pain. As the intervertebral disks age and collapse, the facet joints are loaded with greater forces, hastening the development of degenerative arthritis in these small, posterior spinal articulations. It has been proposed that pain and stiffness that result from facet joint arthritis are a contributing factor to acute and chronic low back discomfort. In reality, it may be that some element of all three conditions (degenerative disk disease, lumbar muscular strain, and posterior element arthritis) is present in these patients.

▶ *Physical Exam*

The yield on physical exam for low back pain (without radiculopathy) is very low. Range-of-motion limits can be meticulously measured, but these measurements are rarely helpful. They may or may not be decreased due to pain. Palpation of the paraspinous muscles may reveal areas of tenderness or even muscle firmness due to spasm. Alternatively, the exam may be completely normal. For the sake of completeness, a physical exam for low back pain should include checking for pain to palpation over the spinous processes and flank percussion. While it is not a particularly sensitive or specific sign, tenderness to palpation over an individual spinous process can indicate the presence of a metastatic vertebral lesion in that vertebra. Pain with flank percussion may indicate a renal cause of the patient's low back pain. The pain may radiate into the buttocks or even the posterior thighs, but true radicular findings such as pain that radiates below the knees, loss of sensation, reflex changes, and motor weakness are absent in these patients who have low back pain without radiculopathy. The examination may be difficult if the patient is very uncomfortable. Weakness due to pain can be confused with weakness secondary to nerve root impingement.

Global weakness that involves multiple muscle groups in the lower extremity is not consistent with a radiculopathy. Figure 6-7

SCIATICA

The sciatic nerve is the peripheral nerve formed by the confluence of the L4, L5, and S1 nerve roots (Figure 6-B). With very few exceptions, the condition we call sciatica results from compression of one of the three nerve roots at the level of the lumbar spine, not from compression of the sciatic nerve itself. If the compression were actually occurring at the level of the sciatic nerve, where all three nerve roots are bundled together, we would see a stocking-like distribution of global numbness, motor weakness, and loss of all reflexes in all three nerve root distributions at the same time. This is rarely, if ever, seen. One example is "pyriformis syndrome." In this condition, a tight contracture of the pyriformis muscle, which crosses over the sciatic nerve at the level of the pelvis, compresses the sciatic nerve.

(continued on following page)

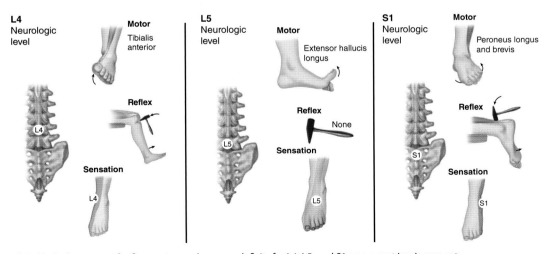

Figure 6-7. Typical patterns of reflex, motor, and sensory deficits for L4, L5, and S1 nerve root impingement.

shows the motor deficits, reflex changes, and patterns of sensory loss one would expect for the most common (L4, L5, and S1) nerve root impingement conditions. In actual clinical practice, weakness due to pain and weakness due to nerve root impingement can be hard to distinguish. The straight leg raise test (Figure 6-8) is a physical exam test used to detect lower lumbar

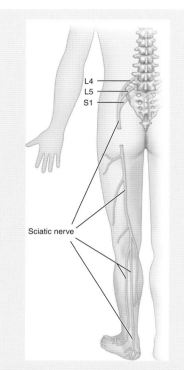

Figure 6-B. The L4, L5, and S1 nerve roots combine to form the sciatic nerve.

This is a very rare condition, and most patients diagnosed with pyriformis syndrome are more likely to have a simple (and much more common) L4, L5, or S1 radiculopathy. Compression of the sciatic nerve along its course from the buttock down the thigh and leg is rare because in its journey down the lower extremity, the nerve and its branches are surrounded by soft, flexible, yielding soft tissue structures. If you hold up the tip of a length of garden hose, letting it hang vertically in front of you, then push against it with the index finger of your other hand, it is very hard to compress it. The hose simply moves out of the way. If you hold it against the wall, you can easily compress the hose between your index finger and the wall. For a disk or other mass to exert a compressive force on

(continued on following page)

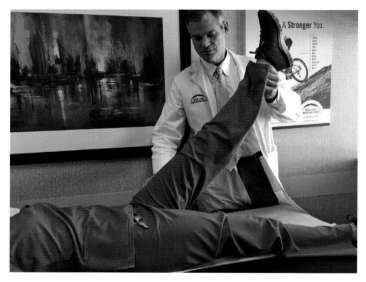

Figure 6-8. The straight leg raise test.

nerve root irritation. The test takes advantage of the fact that, if the knee is locked out straight and the leg is raised, tension is applied to the sciatic nerve. The nerve roots that combine to create the sciatic nerve are the nerve roots most commonly affected by nerve root impingement (L4, L5, and S1), so applying tension to the sciatic nerve applies tension to these nerve roots. If one or more of these nerve roots is significantly inflamed or irritated, this test may elicit pain that radiates down the leg or sensory changes such as numbness, tingling, or electrical sensations. In patients with low back pain only (no radiculopathy), the straight leg raise test may elicit pain in the buttock or posterior thigh, but numbness, tingling, and pain that radiates below the knee are not expected.

▶ Imaging Studies

Anteroposterior (AP) and lateral x-rays of the lumbar spine can show the destructive lesions seen with neoplasm and may show structural abnormalities such as scoliosis, but neoplasms and

provide for their families. Having to miss work is stressful. This stress is compounded by the fact that, unlike those of us trained as medical providers, most patients have not been educated about the typically benign and self-limited natural history of acute low back pain and sciatica.

It is not unusual for a patient who experiences the sudden onset of severe pain, numbness, and weakness to assume that the condition could evolve into full-blown paralysis. While we know that absent neoplasm, infection, or high-energy trauma, paralysis is essentially unheard of, the average patient does not. It is helpful to take the time to explain that, when a disk herniation occurs, much of the pressure compressing the adjacent nerve root is the result of acute inflammation, which subsides over time. Also, the disk material that has herniated into the spinal canal can, and often does, resorb (Figure 6-14). Sharing this information and images like the ones in Figure 6-14 can help us reassure our patients more effectively.

Before...

...9 months later

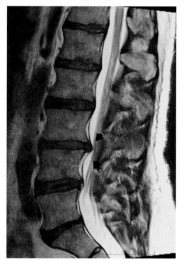
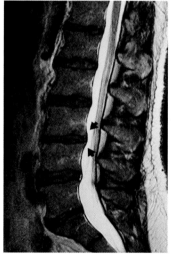

Figure 6-14. An MRI image showing a lumbar disk herniation (arrows). After 9 months with no treatment other than the passage of time, the disk herniation has resolved.

▶ *Surgical Treatment*

While surgical procedures exist to decompress the nerve root impingement caused by disk extrusions and herniations, the literature lacks well-designed studies proving their superiority over nonoperative treatment. Surgery is typically reserved for patients with recalcitrant symptoms or progressive neurologic deficits, and even in these patients, the efficacy of surgical intervention is a matter of controversy and debate.

then sections of the laminae and posterior elements are removed to increase the volume of the spinal canal. This operation is known as a laminectomy and decompression (Figures 6-D and 6-E).

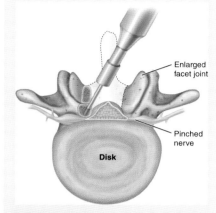

Figure 6-D. Lumbar decompression surgery for foraminal spinal stenosis involves widening the passages in the spine through which the nerve roots pass.

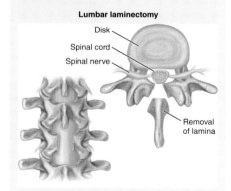

Figure 6-E. Lumbar decompression surgery for central spinal stenosis involves removing the posterior wall of the spinal canal by excising all or part of the laminae. This increases the volume of the canal.

There is no surgical procedure for muscular low back pain, but back pain

(continued on following page)

caused by arthritis can be treated with either a fusion or a disk replacement operation. In arthritis, pain results from bone-on-bone articulation. This can occur anteriorly, if the intervertebral disks have deteriorated and adjacent vertebral bodies are malarticulating, or posteriorly, if the facet joints become arthritic. In the fusion operation, pain from bone-on-bone articulation is eliminated by rigidly bonding (fusing) adjacent vertebrae together. The vertebrae are fused by surgically exposing the posterior elements and bridging the gap between the two vertebrae with a bone graft. The bone graft heals to the two vertebrae to create a solid vertebrae–bone graft–vertebrae structure. If multiple levels are fused (Figure 6-F), the surgeon may add metal

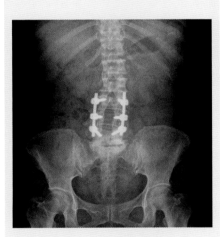

Figure 6-F. A two-level lumbar spinal fusion. The rods and screws immobilize the levels that are being fused. Bone graft is used to create a solid bone bridge connecting adjacent vertebrae (*Licensed from Shutterstock*).

rods, screws, or plates to help solidify the fusion. Any time a part of a mobile section of the skeleton is fused, the adjacent sections move more to compensate; consequently, those adjacent sections are subject to higher forces, stresses, and

(continued on following page)

LOW BACK PAIN *WITH* RADICULOPATHY: SPINAL STENOSIS

In addition to displaced disk material, arthritis of the lumbar spine can lead to the development of radicular signs and symptoms. Arthritis is a productive process. It stimulates the overproduction of synovial fluid, bone (osteophytes/bone spurs), and hypertrophic synovial soft tissue. Figure 6-15 shows a familiar example

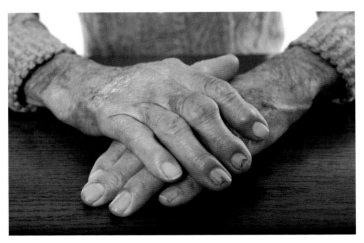

Figure 6-15. An example of joint enlargement due to arthritis (*Licensed from Shutterstock*).

of the joint enlargement that is typically associated with arthritis. In the condition known as spinal stenosis, arthritic enlargement of the facet joints and posterior elements of the spine causes a mass effect that can compress the lumbar nerve roots. Spinal stenosis can occur in the neural foramina (foraminal stenosis), the central spinal canal (central stenosis), or both.

Spinal stenosis is typically a problem of older patients. These arthritic anatomic changes are common in older patients and are thought to be present in up to a third of people over the age of 60, though only a minority of them will become symptomatic. The classic history for a patient with spinal stenosis of the lumbar spine is that of pain that radiates from the buttocks distally into the legs, and typically it is made worse with standing or walking. This presentation is so classic for spinal stenosis that it has been given a special name: *neurogenic claudication*.

Neurogenic claudication shares some of the same features of vascular claudication, and, to confuse matters, the two can coexist in the same patient. Differentiating factors include the fact that, in neurogenic claudication, the pain typically starts proximally and radiates distally, whereas in vascular claudication, the pain starts distally and radiates proximally. Furthermore, patients with vascular claudication receive relief if they stop walking and stand, while patients with neurogenic claudication do not get relief with standing and have to sit or lean forward to alleviate their symptoms. Sitting and leaning forward help relieve the symptoms of spinal stenosis because the dimensions of the spinal canal and foramina *increase* with forward flexion and *decrease* with extension. This is shown in Figure 6-16. A classic symptom of lumbar spinal stenosis

strains. With time, patients with lumbar fusions are likely to experience degenerative changes at adjacent levels, and many of them eventually require additional operations to extend their fusions to include adjacent vertebrae. The artificial lumbar disk replacement operation was introduced as an alternative to lumbar fusion (Figure 6-G). The operation is

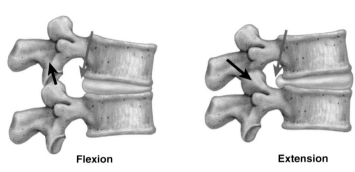

Flexion   **Extension**

Figure 6-16. Forward flexion of the lumbar spine increases the dimensions of the lumbar spinal canal and foramina; extension of the lumbar spine decreases the dimensions of these neural passageways.

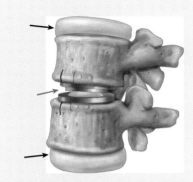

Figure 6-G. The artificial disk replacement (red arrow).

is the "shopping cart sign." Patients will find themselves leaning over onto the shopping cart as they grocery shop. This flexes the spine and relieves their symptoms. In severe cases of spinal stenosis, patients may develop subtle bladder and bowel symptoms, but in older patients (the demographic most likely to have spinal stenosis) prostate disease and stress incontinence are common and can be hard to differentiate from neurogenic symptoms.

relatively new, and high-quality, long-term data are still being collected, but because it preserves motion, it is hoped that the incidence of adjacent-level disease will be lower in patients treated with disk replacements than in those who underwent spinal fusion.

▶ *Physical Exam*

As is the case with the other conditions we have discussed in this chapter, the physical exam is not always that helpful. Back pain and stiffness are common findings, but not specific to the diagnosis of spinal stenosis. Leg pain and weakness precipitated by exertion on a treadmill (especially if it resolves with forward flexion) is a compelling physical exam finding, but not always practical in an office setting. Checking peripheral pulses can help to differentiate spinal stenosis from vascular claudication, but asymptomatic age-related atherosclerosis often makes peripheral pulses weak and hard to find in patients in this age group. The spine is a common target for metastatic disease, so deep, firm palpation of the spinous processes to elicit the focal, localized tenderness seen with a vertebral metastatic lesion should be a part of the exam. The exam may demonstrate subtle lower extremity weakness, but this may be hard to differentiate from weakness related

BONE TUMOR BASICS

Question: What is the most common neoplasm of bone?

Answer: A metastatic lesion.

Question: What are the primary neoplasms that commonly metastasize to bone?

Answer: Breast, lung, renal, prostate, and thyroid.

Question: What is the most common *primary* neoplasm of bone?

Answer: Multiple myeloma.

IS THAT ALL YOU'VE GOT?

Treating patients with low back pain issues can be a difficult task. Evidence-based medicine has little to offer, other than the reassurance that the majority of patients improve with time. Unfortunately, "time" can mean 3-6 months, and, after resolution of an acute episode, recurrence rates are high. We may be able to allay their fears of permanent nerve damage, chronic debilitating pain, paralysis, and disability with emotional support and education. A few days of rest combined with a short course of NSAIDs may help them through the initial, severe discomfort they experience. But, the second phase of a strictly evidence-based

(continued on following page)

age, inactivity, or pain. Sensory deficits can be seen with spinal stenosis, and diminished ankle and knee reflexes may be present as well, although the absence of brisk reflexes can simply be age related. Hyperreflexia can result from severe spinal stenosis with myelopathy, especially in cases of canal stenosis of the thoracic and cervical spine. The straight leg raise sign, most helpful in the physical exam for patients with disk herniations, may or may not be positive in patients with spinal stenosis.

▶ *Imaging Studies*

Plain films and more sophisticated imaging studies like MRI or computed tomographic (CT) scans can help to rule out metastatic disease. These studies will likely demonstrate the arthritic changes seen with spinal stenosis, but, again, arthritic changes are commonplace in older patients, and their significance in making the diagnosis of spinal stenosis is limited.

▶ *Medical Treatment*

As its name implies, spinal stenosis is a problem of decreased dimensions, specifically, decreased dimensions of the neural passageways in the bones of the spine. Arthritic bone spurs (osteophytes) create dimensional changes that are static and typically do not change with time (other than the gradual increase in their size that accompanies the progression of arthritis seen with aging). Synovial hypertrophy and the overproduction of synovial fluid in small articulations, like the facet joints of the lumbar spine, are dynamic and may increase and decrease depending on the level of local inflammation. NSAIDs, oral corticosteroids, and epidural steroid injections are intended to decrease inflammation in an attempt to mitigate the dynamic component of nerve compression seen in spinal stenosis. Their therapeutic value is not supported by high-level clinical studies, and their use in the treatment of spinal stenosis is controversial, but many feel that they can be very helpful. The value of physical therapy is also a matter of contentious debate. Exercises that emphasize lumbar flexion strength and decrease lumbar extension posture have been advocated by some, and a fitness program designed to decrease or eliminate unnecessary intra-abdominal fat to facilitate forward flexion of the lumbar spine make sense empirically, but data to support them are lacking.

▶ *Surgical Treatment*

The operations designed to address lumbar spinal stenosis all involve removing bone from the central canal or neural foramina to increase their dimensions and decompress the involved nerve roots. Surgical intervention, if indicated, should be reserved for patients who have failed conservative treatment or have progressive neurologic deficits. Surgically exposing the lumbar spine involves dissecting away important muscle attachments and inevitably results in some degree of consequent muscle injury, and removing bone from aged, arthritic vertebrae can destabilize the spine. The data supporting decompression operations for lumbar spinal stenosis are more convincing and more accepted than those for any other type of back surgery, but the indications, efficacy, and therapeutic value of these procedures remain controversial and debated.

CRITICAL CONDITIONS OF THE LUMBAR SPINE

Overall, the incidence of critical spinal conditions, especially in an office setting where spinal trauma is not likely a consideration, is exceedingly low. Unfortunately, things that are rare are also easy to miss, and the sequelae of missed critical spinal conditions are usually grave. The specter of irreversible neurologic damage, paralysis, permanent bowel and bladder dysfunction, and other consequences of certain spinal conditions incite fear and unrest among patients and providers alike. Infection, hematoma, neoplasm, and critical spinal instability account for almost all of the dangerous spinal conditions we are likely to encounter in our patients. While atraumatic critical instability of the cervical spine can be seen as a result of the destructive changes associated with rheumatoid arthritis, this condition is almost unheard of in the lumbar spine. Constitutional symptoms such as fever, chills, night sweats, and weight loss may indicate infection or neoplasm. In the spine, neoplasm is most likely metastatic disease, and there are certain cancers that typically metastasize to bone (see sidebar, page 190). Severe, intractable pain, rapidly progressive neurologic changes, gait disturbances, night pain, and the loss of the ability to ambulate are all "red flags," as are dramatic changes in bowel or bladder function.

The single best test to evaluate a patient suspected of having a critical spinal condition is an MRI. The MRI is an excellent study for identifying the location and extent of an epidural abscess, hematoma, or spinal neoplasm, and it can also demonstrate structural changes associated with critical instability, although flexion and extension imaging may be needed to more thoroughly assess instability. The treatment of spinal neoplasms is lesion specific and may or may not require immediate attention, but making the diagnosis and promptly initiating treatment of the primary has obvious benefits in the treatment of almost every type of cancer. Expeditious evaluation and treatment of critical instability and infection and hematoma are essential if permanent nerve injury is to be avoided or, at least, minimized.

treatment plan, which is limited to an exercise program that emphasizes a review of proper lifting mechanics and aerobic fitness, doesn't always meet our patient's expectations. The only tips that I can offer for patients wading through the "doldrums" of an episode of low back pain (and I have to emphasize that these are anecdotal, not evidence based, and not always that helpful) are as follows:

1. Do everything you can to try to avoid prescribing narcotic pain medication. Symptoms can take months to resolve, and, over that period of time, chronic narcotic use can lead to habituation and addiction.

2. Check in with patients frequently. Something as simple as a phone call can mean a lot to a patient who feels helpless and is in pain.

3. Make changes. Try different things. Recommend a different NSAID. Suggest they alternate their NSAID with acetaminophen. Change their exercises. These changes may not make much of a difference medically, but the fact that you are checking in with them, listening to what they have to say, and adjusting things conveys a message that you are engaged, interested, and involved. This is an important message for someone in desperate straights who is having to "wait it out" until their condition improves. The last thing a patient in this situation needs is to feel neglected, ignored, or "blown-off."

4. Be open-minded when patients pursue unorthodox treatment. There are a limitless number of treatments that lack what would be considered, strictly speaking, "strong medical evidence." Acupuncture, chiropractic treatment, massage, Rolfing, reiki, magnets, lasers, special belts, special pillows, traction apparatuses, heating pads, cooling pads, meditation, braces,

(continued on following page)

creams, salves, reflexology, the list goes on and on. While randomized, controlled clinical trials proving the efficacy of many of these treatments may remain elusive, there is a body of anecdotal evidence for each of them, and some patients do respond. Or do they? Many patients will try a number of these treatments during the course of their recovery. They may get better as the result of time alone, but whichever treatment they are using when they finally feel better appears to them to be curative. The statistics are excellent that these patients will get better in 3 to 6 months. Our job is to get them there. For patients with radicular symptoms, I will occasionally resort to an epidural steroid injection. The meta-analysis data indicate that the benefits of epidural steroid injections, if they exist at all, are short lived. They may only give relief for a few months. I'm OK with that. If I can give a frustrated, desperate patient a few months of relief over the course of a 3- to 6-month recovery, that works for me. I will often use an in-office epidural steroid injection technique in which the medication is injected into the epidural space using the sacral hiatus. This technique is not quite as effective as an x-ray–guided, transforaminal injection, but is much, much less expensive and much more convenient for the patient. The total cost for the medication, injection equipment (needle, syringe, prep), and professional fee for administering the injection (CPT code 62322) is less than $100. The technique for an in-office epidural injection is described in Chapter 9.

5. Avoid the sirens' song. Opting for a surgical solution can be tempting for a patient in the doldrums. Patients need to understand that we may have a *surgery* for them, but we don't have a *surgical solution* for them.

CHRONIC BACK PAIN

While the majority of patients with an acute episode of low back pain will become better over the course of 3 to 6 months, a few will not. For these unfortunate patients, low back pain can become a chronic condition. The treatment of chronic low back pain is fraught with disappointments and failure. Expectations must be modest, and cures are rare. Successful treatment may be defined as developing a strategy to cope with the pain and disability while preserving the ability to function in society. With the proper education, interest, and office infrastructure, you may choose to manage these patients with chronic pain on your own. Alternatively, you may elect to recruit the assistance of a pain management specialist, if such a resource exists in your community (see sidebar (Page 190)).

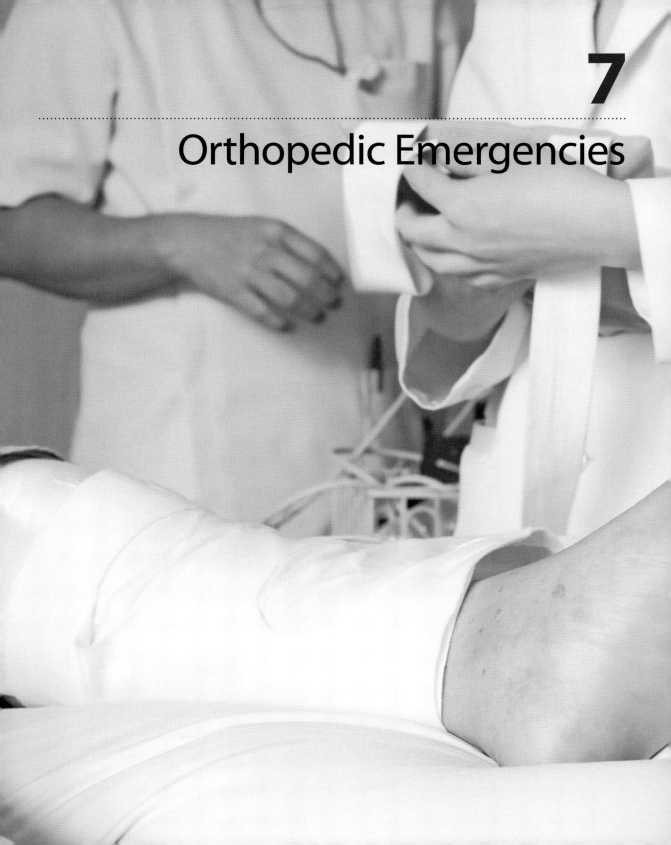

7

Orthopedic Emergencies

Merriam-Webster defines an emergency as "an unexpected and usually dangerous situation that calls for immediate action." Most outpatient clinic visits, especially *orthopedic* outpatient clinic visits, do not fall into this category. Outpatient orthopedic conditions are rarely dangerous and seldom require immediate action, so encountering an orthopedic emergency in an outpatient setting would certainly be "unexpected." But, it can, and does, happen, and missing an orthopedic emergency can have devastating consequences. This chapter is intended to arm primary care providers with the knowledge they need to identify orthopedic emergencies when they see them and to give them a strategy for dealing with orthopedic emergencies in those rare instances when they might present in an outpatient setting.

Let's start with two orthopedic emergencies you'll likely never see outside the emergency room but are common enough to deserve a few lines of explanation in the chapter.

EXTREMITY AMPUTATIONS

Acute, traumatic toe and (more commonly) finger amputations are injuries you may never see but may well encounter in the form of a panicked phone call from a hysterical patient who hasn't thought things through enough to just head straight to the nearest emergency room. The instructions for this patient are simple:

1. **Call 911 and request an ambulance for expedient transport to the nearest emergency department.** It is not recommended that these patients drive themselves to the emergency room as blood loss and shock may impair reaction time and judgment or even result in a loss of consciousness.
2. **Do not eat or drink anything.** If the digit is to be surgically reimplanted, immediate surgery is necessary, and an empty stomach makes general anesthesia much safer.
3. **Wrap the amputated digit in a clean, moist cloth and place it in a plastic bag.** Seal the bag and place it in a second bag filled with ice. Cooling the amputated part will prolong its viability and increase the odds that the reimplantation will succeed.

INJURIES THAT RESULT IN AN UNSTABLE SPINE

Any patient with severe neck or back pain after significant trauma may have an unstable spine. Displacement of an unstable spine can result in spinal cord or nerve root injury and permanent neurologic impairment. "Severe pain" and "significant trauma" are subjective criteria, which can make diagnosing an unstable spine difficult. It is prudent to err on the side of caution. If there is any doubt or if the patient is complaining of neurologic symptoms (numbness, tingling, weakness), the patient should be evaluated in the emergency department with either flexion/extension x-rays or a magnetic resonance imaging (MRI) of the spine.

POST-TRAUMATIC COMPARTMENT SYNDROME

Post-traumatic compartment syndrome is a rapidly evolving, potentially devastating complication of blunt injury to an extremity. Crush injuries can result in compartment syndrome as well. In the extremities, muscle groups are contained in thick, dense envelopes of fascia called compartments. While this condition can develop in the thighs, arms, and forearms, the fascial compartments are thickest in the legs, so compartment syndrome is most common there. Figure 7-1 shows three separate muscle groups in three individual compartments.

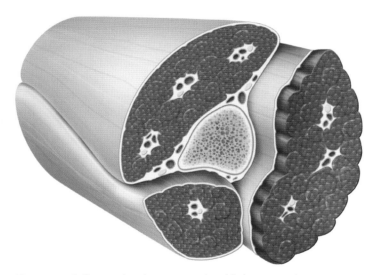

Figure 7-1. A diagram showing an extremity with three separate compartments.

Figure 7-2 shows a schematic representation of the circulatory system of a typical muscle compartment. The compartment, a pink square in the diagram, is bordered by four black lines representing the dense, noncompliant fascial walls that envelope the compartment. The illustration shows a single, large-diameter artery bringing blood into the compartment. Blood entering the compartment through this artery is under relatively high pressure. If the patient's blood pressure is 120/80 mm Hg, the mean pressure

BUILDING A COMPARTMENT PRESSURE-MEASUREMENT TOOL

Materials needed:

1. A blood pressure manometer
2. Intravenous tubing with a three-way stopcock
3. A 20-mL syringe
4. An 18-gauge, 1.5-inch long needle

Instructions:

A. Attach the syringe to the three-way stopcock as shown in Figure 7-A. Attach one end of the intravenous tubing to a blood pressure manometer and the other end to an 18-gauge needle.

B. Close the three-way stopcock to the manometer and draw a small amount of saline into the tubing. Draw enough saline into the tubing so that the saline fills the tubing up to a point just before reaching the three-way stopcock (red arrow).

C. Open all three ports of the three-way stop cock.

D. Prep the patient's skin and insert the needle into the compartment to be measured.

E. Slowly depress the plunger on the syringe as you watch the place on the intravenous tubing where the column of saline ends. As you depress the plunger on the syringe, the pressure in the tubing will rise, and this will be reflected by a rise in the pressure reading on the manometer. If the column of saline is creeping up the tubing toward the three-way stopcock, then the pressure in the compartment

(continued on following page)

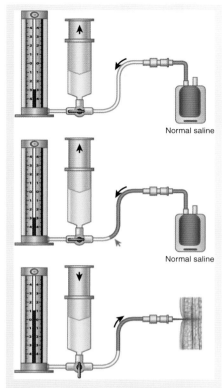

Figure 7-A. Building your own compartment pressure measuring device.

is higher than the pressure applied by the syringe. As you increase the pressure by pressing harder on the plunger of the syringe, there will be a point at which the column of saline stops moving. At this point, the pressure generated by the syringe is equal to the pressure of the compartment. If you continue to press even harder, the pressure in the tubing will exceed the compartment pressure and the column of saline will start to creep *down* the tubing, toward the patient.

F. Record the reading registered on the gauge of the manometer at the pressure where the column of saline was not moving in either direction. That is the compartment pressure.

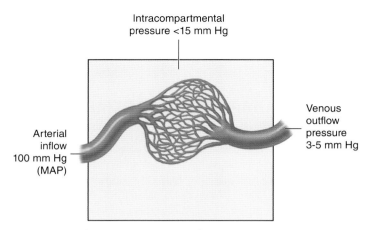

Figure 7-2. A schematic representation of a compartment. Note the high-pressure arterial inflow and low-pressure venous outflow.

in this artery is 100 mm Hg. Once it enters the compartment, this artery branches into arterioles, which terminate as small-diameter capillaries that are the site of the nutrient and oxygen/carbon dioxide exchange that keep the muscles in the compartment alive. These capillaries combine to form veinules, which coalesce, in this model, into a single, large-diameter vein that allows blood to exit the compartment. The typical pressure inside the compartment is less than 15 mm Hg, and the pressure inside the large-diameter vein is about 3-5 mm Hg. It is the pressure gradient between the high-pressure arterial inflow vessel and the low-pressure venous outflow vessel that drives blood through the compartment.

Blunt or crush trauma that is sufficient to tear the high-pressure vessels on the arterial side but does not lacerate the fascial boundaries of the compartment sets the stage for the development of compartment syndrome. The key is that the trauma is blunt, and that the closed system of the compartment remains intact. Deep lacerations that split open the fascia abolish the closed system of the compartment and make the development of compartment syndrome impossible.

In compartment syndrome, blood from the ruptured, high-pressure artery or arteriole will continue to flow from the injured vessel into the relatively low-pressure compartment space until the pressure inside the compartment reaches that of the arterial blood supply. As the compartment pressure rises, a sequence of devastating consequences ensues. First, the compartment pressure reaches a level high enough to cause collapse of the walls of the low-pressure outflow vessels on the venous side. This results in the stasis of blood flow and muscle tissue ischemia. As the muscle cells in the compartment become ischemic and die, they lyse and release their cytoplasm, resulting in an increase in the osmotic pressure of the extracellular space inside the compartment, favoring the development of even higher compartment pressures. These heightened pressures cause additional injury and death to the muscles, nerves, and other tissues within the compartment. Before long, irreversible tissue damage has occurred, and the extremity is permanently compromised.

Clearly, the most important aspect of the management of compartment syndrome is to recognize and treat the condition before irreversible damage has occurred. A history of high-energy, blunt or crushing trauma may be the most important clue. If you are evaluating a patient who has multiple fractures in a single extremity, like the patient whose x-ray is shown in Figure 7-3, and

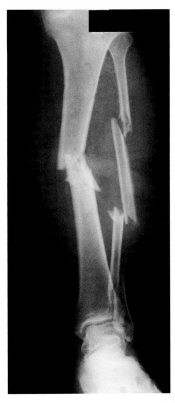

Figure 7-3. An x-ray of the tibia and fibula suggesting a high-energy extremity injury. If there is no associated laceration and the compartments are intact, this is the type of injury that can lead to the development of compartment syndrome (*Licensed from Shutterstock*).

there is no associated laceration, then you must keep the possibility of compartment syndrome in mind. Other signs and symptoms include (1) pain that is out of proportion to the injury; (2) a firm, swollen, tense extremity; and (3) pain with passive motion of the distal parts.

Testing for pain with passive motion of the distal parts takes advantage of the fact that many of the muscles that control our toes and fingers are located in our legs and forearms, respectively. They move our digits using a system of long, slender tendons, much like the strings that are used to move a string puppet (see the sidebar in Chapter 4, page 126, for more details). If you gently flex and extend a patient's finger or toe, you are alternately pulling on the flexor and extensor tendons and proximal muscle bellies attached to those tendons, causing them to move back and forth in their muscle compartments. If the compartment in which the muscles reside is experiencing compartment syndrome, this will be excruciatingly painful.

Other signs and symptoms of compartment syndrome include the "4 Ps" (pain, pallor, paresthesias, and pulselessness). While these four findings are certainly present in most cases of compartment syndrome, they occur late in the course of the condition. It would be best to make the diagnosis before these findings present so that treatment can be initiated before irreversible tissue damage has occurred.

One tool that can be useful in making the diagnosis early is a compartment pressure-measuring instrument (Figure 7-4). These

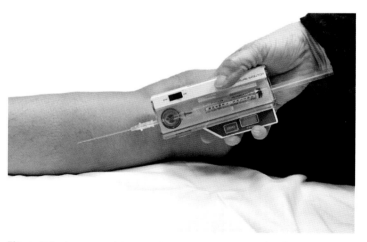

Figure 7-4. A commercial compartment pressure-measuring device.

are commercially available and are standard equipment in most emergency departments. Alternatively, if you are in your office or another location where such an instrument is not available, you can build one yourself using a blood pressure manometer, intravenous tubing, a syringe, and a three-way stopcock (see sidebar, page 195).

The pressure should be measured with the needle deep in the muscle of the suspected compartment. A map of the compartments in the leg is shown in Figure 7-5. The pressure in a normal,

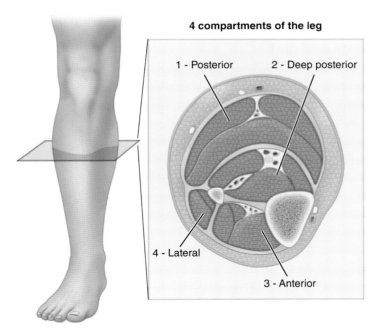

4 compartments of the leg

1 - Posterior   2 - Deep posterior

4 - Lateral

3 - Anterior

Figure 7-5. The four compartments of the leg. The leg is the most common location for compartment syndrome because the fascial envelopes that surround the muscles of the leg are firm, strong, and inelastic.

resting compartment should be less than 15 mm Hg. If the muscles in the compartment have been recently exercised, pressures up to 30 mm Hg are considered normal. Pressures over 45 mm Hg are considered to be diagnostic of compartment syndrome. Patients with compartment pressures between 30 and 45 mm Hg should be monitored carefully. Acute, post-traumatic compartment syndrome evolves quickly. Repeating compartment pressure measurements every 20 minutes for 2 hours should reveal an evolving compartment syndrome.

▶ Treatment

There is no medical treatment for compartment syndrome. If the patient has a coagulopathy that is causing bleeding within the compartment, that coagulopathy should be addressed. Also, be aware of rhabdomyolysis, which often accompanies compartment syndrome due to large volumes of dead muscle tissue. Aggressive hydration may be needed to avoid renal injury.

The only treatment that can arrest the tissue damage caused by compartment syndrome is a surgical compartment release (Figure 7-6). In this procedure, the fascial envelope that is the wall of the compartment is incised and split wide open from top to bottom, releasing the pressure in the compartment and abolishing the closed system that is required to create compartment syndrome.

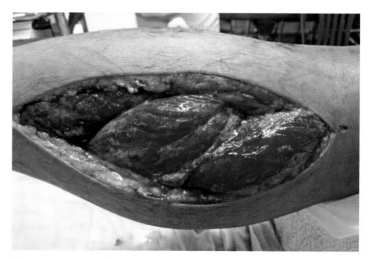

Figure 7-6. An open fasciotomy. This procedure splits the compartment wide open, from top to bottom, abolishing the closed system and eliminating elevated compartment pressures (*Licensed from Shutterstock*).

In most cases, the swollen, ischemic muscle herniates out through the fascial incision, making it impossible to close the skin. After 2-3 days, the muscle edema typically subsides, and a second surgery is required to debride necrotic muscle and close the wound.

NEUROVASCULAR INJURIES ASSOCIATED WITH EXTREMITY FRACTURES AND DISLOCATIONS

Figure 7-7 shows one of the most common fractures in all of orthopedics: the Colles fracture. When a patient falls on their

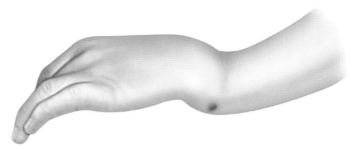

Figure 7-7. A Colles fracture deformity. This deformity can kink the neurovascular structures on the volar side of the wrist, resulting in neurovascular compromise. Typically, the neurovascular compromise associated with this injury resolves once the fracture is reduced and the deformity corrected.

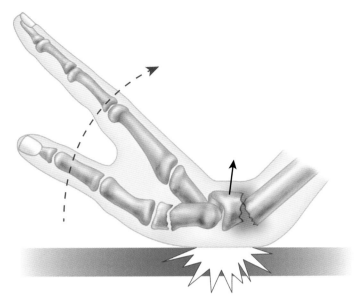

Figure 7-8. The Colles fracture: A fall onto the outstretched hand fractures the distal radius. The distal portion of the fractured radius displaces dorsally (black arrow), producing the classic deformity seen in Figure 7-7.

outstretched hand, the distal radius typically fractures in the pattern depicted in Figure 7-8, creating the deformity seen in Figure 7-7. All of the important neurovascular structures (the median and ulnar nerves and the radial and ulnar arteries) reside on the anterior (volar) side of the forearm, wrist, and palm, and they can be "tented" or stretched over the broken end of the shaft of the radius (Figure 7-9). Similarly, the deformity created by a dislocation can kink neurovascular structures. Deforming the nerves and arteries in this way can result in their malfunction and, potentially, long-term consequences.

For that reason, it is important to perform a neurovascular evaluation any time you are evaluating a patient with an orthopedic injury to an extremity. Be sure to document your findings. If, for example, the circulation in an injured extremity is compromised and you apply a splint, reduce the fracture, or intervene in any other way, it is important to document that the circulatory issue existed *before* your intervention. Otherwise, you may be blamed for causing it. Fortunately, the neurovascular structures in most orthopedic fractures and dislocations are rarely torn or lacerated, and function returns once the deformity is corrected. This is amazing, considering how sharp and jagged the fracture fragments appear on x-ray.

In this chapter, we discuss nerve and vascular injuries separately. Let's start with nerve injuries associated with traumatic

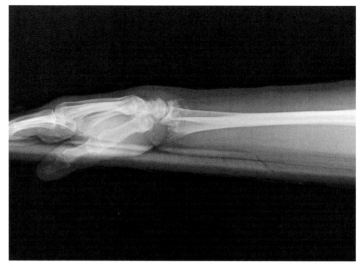

A

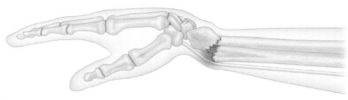

B

Figure 7-9. The x-ray in **A** shows the deformity typical of a displaced Colles fracture. (*Image licensed from Shutterstock*) The illustration in **B** shows how this deformity can kink the volar neurovascular structures. Similar fracture or dislocation deformities elsewhere in the musculoskeletal system can create neurovascular compromise as well.

deformities, and let's continue to use the Colles fracture as an example. The neurologic examination of an injured extremity is a limited assessment of nerve function. The nerves in our extremities have motor, sensory, and autonomic functions. Assessing autonomic function is not practical in this setting, and motor function assessments are difficult to perform due to the pain patients experience when they move muscles attached to fractured bones. For these reasons, we are limited to using the evaluation of sensation as an index of nerve function. Many different methods exist for assessing sensation, but the ability to feel light touch is sufficient and requires no special equipment or training. Be sure to measure and document the grade of sensation (normal, subjectively decreased, or absent) and the location (e.g., "median nerve distribution" or "dorsum of all five fingers").

▶ Treatment

As mentioned, it is exceedingly rare for a nerve to be torn or lacerated by the fracture fragments. In most cases, the sensory deficit will resolve once the fracture deformity is corrected. If you are comfortable attempting to reduce the fracture yourself, then proceed as soon as the initial neurovascular assessment is completed. In many cases, you may not feel comfortable reducing the fracture. If that is the case, then it is important to expedite the patient into the care of someone who can. You are never "required" to perform a procedure that you do not feel comfortable performing. If you live in a rural area and the closest orthopedic provider is many hours away, so by the time the patient arrives there permanent nerve damage has occurred, that is unfortunate, but it is not substandard medical care. Your responsibility is to recognize the deficit, understand that it constitutes an emergency, and do your best to have the patient treated as soon as possible.

If you do correct the deformity, the next step is to repeat the sensory exam. In most cases, the neurologic deficit will resolve relatively quickly once the pressure that the fracture fragment is applying to the nerve has been removed. Be sure to document the results of this second sensory exam as well. If the sensory exam normalizes, then a splint to maintain the corrected position of the fracture is usually the next step. If you attempt to correct the deformity but are unsuccessful and the deformity persists after your attempt, consult an orthopedic specialist immediately. In some cases, correction may require an open reduction/internal fixation surgical procedure. If the sensory deficit does not improve after the fracture deformity has been successfully corrected, no immediate action is required. The extremity should be splinted and orthopedic follow-up within 1 week should be arranged (see sidebar for an explanation).

VASCULAR INJURIES

The radial and ulnar arteries and their branches nourish the hand and fingers. Like the median and ulnar nerves, these structures are located on the volar side of the wrist and can be occluded if they are kinked by a fracture deformity. Similarly, arteries elsewhere in the extremities are susceptible to occlusion when adjacent fractures or dislocations deform them. We are less concerned with venous occlusion. The arterial and venous circulatory systems differ in many ways, one of which is that blood is delivered to our extremities by a few, large-diameter arteries and returned to the heart by a network of many, many smaller-caliber veins. Occluding a major vein may result in venous congestion, but it will not completely arrest the venous circulation; blood will simply return through the other remaining veins. If, however, a major artery is occluded, the tissues that are nourished by that artery are at risk for ischemia and death.

WHAT?!? WE'RE SENDING A PATIENT HOME WITH A NEUROLOGIC DEFICIT AFTER A FRACTURE?!?

In the discussion of the treatment of a neurologic deficit associated with a fracture or dislocation deformity, it is recommended that sensory deficits that don't resolve after reduction of the fracture and correction of the deformity be observed and followed on an elective basis. How does that make any sense? The same neurologic deficit that was an emergency before the fracture was reduced is now considered not to be an emergency? Why?

To understand the explanation, we need to review the three different types of nerve injury: neuropraxia, axonotmesis, and neurotmesis. Neuropraxia is the least severe of the three types of injury. In neuropraxia, there is loss of nerve function without structural damage to the nerve. Neuropraxia is usually the result of ischemia (see the discussion of neuropraxia as it relates to peripheral nerve entrapment conditions in the sidebar in Chapter 4, page 116). When nerves around a fracture are "kinked" by the fracture deformity, the pressure on the nerve temporarily interrupts its blood supply (just like the skin on your palm blanches when you press hard on it with your fingertip). Correcting the fracture deformity and removing the kink in the nerve is the equivalent of taking your finger off your palm. Blood flow to the nerve is restored, and function returns. In some cases of neuropraxia, the myelin sheaths that insulate the intact nerve axons are damaged, and healing can take days or weeks.

Axonotmesis is the term used to describe an injury in which the axons in the nerve are destroyed, but the epineurium (the tough fibrous sheath that forms the outer "skin" of the nerve) remains intact (Figure 7-B). After an axonotmesis injury, the structural damage

(continued on following page)

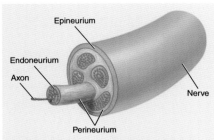

Figure 7-B. An illustration of the cross-sectional anatomy of a peripheral nerve.

to the nerve must heal before function can return. A signal that disruption of the axon has occurred makes its way up the uninjured section of the axon to the nerve's cell body. All of the organelles needed for protein synthesis are located in the cell body, which, in some cases, is several feet away from the place on the axon where repair is needed. Materials synthesized in the cell body are then transported down the axon to the site of injury by a network of microtubules that run like railroad tracks down the length of the axon. The section of the axon distal to the injury dies and disintegrates, leaving empty, hollow endoneurial tubes down which the sprouting new axons can grow.

This process is called Wallerian degeneration. The axon is rebuilt from the site of injury distally, all the way down to the nerve terminus. This process takes time. It may take as long as 2 weeks for the signal of injury to reach the cell body, for protein synthesis to start, and for the first building materials to finally reach the site of injury. The sprouting axon tip will grow at a rate of about a millimeter a day (approximately an inch a month), so recovery of nerve function may take several months. In some instances, several months may be too long.

At the end of every peripheral nerve axon is a specialized end organ. For motor nerve axons, this end organ is the motor end plate, the interface between the end of the nerve and the muscle

(continued on following page)

The vascular surgeons have a term they call the *warm ischemia time*, which is the time after which tissue undergoes irreversible damage due to lack of arterial blood supply. This time is inversely proportionate to the tissue's metabolic rate, which is in turn proportionate to the tissue temperature. The lower the tissue temperature, the longer that tissue can tolerate ischemia. At 98.6 degrees Fahrenheit, the warm ischemia time for human tissue is on the order of 4 hours. This means that, if you are evaluating an injured extremity and pulses are absent, arterial blood flow must be reestablished within 4 hours to avoid irreversible damage.

We mentioned previously that, when assessing the neurologic status of an injured extremity, we use sensation as a surrogate indicator for nerve function. Similarly, when we evaluate the vascular status of an injured extremity, we actually only measure arterial function, which is only a part of the overall vascular status. Our "neurovascular exam" would be more accurately described as an "arterosensory exam." Typically, we use the presence or absence of an arterial pulse as an index of circulatory system function. Measuring the radial and ulnar pulses for injuries in the proximal upper extremity works well, and measuring the dorsalis pedis and posterior tibial pulses works well for proximal injuries to the lower extremity, but measuring arterial function in a distal extremity injury can be challenging. It is often the case in the distal extremities (where many of these injuries occur) that these vessels are too small to allow for a palpable pulse. In the example of our Colles fracture, for instance, the pulses we would need to assess would be in the digital arteries along the medial and lateral sides of the fingers, and these pulses can be hard to palpate. A Doppler device can be helpful in these situations, and if such a device is not available, then pallor, temperature, and capillary refill are probably the best tools for making this assessment. A pale, cool hand with poor capillary refill in the tips of the fingers would suggest an arterial occlusion.

Fortunately, as is the case for the nerve injuries described previously, the vast majority of the arterial occlusions that result from orthopedic injury deformities are completely reversible. Correcting the deformity and "unkinking" the artery restores robust blood flow in almost every case. As is the case with nerve injuries, an extremity with arterial occlusion is an emergency. The clock is running, and, in the case of arterial occlusion, we only have a few hours *from the time of the injury* to restore arterial flow. It is critical that these injuries be recognized immediately and an attempt to reduce the deformity initiated as soon as possible.

Again, if you do not feel comfortable correcting the deformity yourself, you are not obliged to do so, but you are obliged to recognize that this is an emergency and contact a provider who is comfortable performing the procedure. Cooling the extremity can buy more time, but take care not to injure the extremity by applying ice directly to the skin. Wrap the extremity at risk in a moist cloth, then apply ice around the cloth. Be sure to document the neurovascular status before and after any attempt to reduce the fracture or dislocation. If you attempt to correct the deformity but are unsuccessful and the arterial occlusion persists after your attempt, consult an orthopedic specialist immediately. Correction may require an open reduction/internal fixation procedure. If you are successful in correcting the deformity, but the circulatory exam does not normalize (this is rare), then notify a vascular specialist immediately. Typically, the vascular surgeon will ask for an arteriogram to better localize the area of occlusion, and this can often be done in the time it takes for the vascular surgeon to arrive. In most instances, a thrombus or an intimal tear of the arterial wall is the cause of the persistent occlusion, and these lesions can often be treated with transluminal techniques. Occasionally, the artery is transected, and a repair or bypass is required.

SEPTIC ARTHRITIS

The preservation of healthy articular cartilage is a critical part of orthopedic patient care. Once damaged, this important material does not heal or regenerate, and without it, joint function suffers significantly (see Chapter 1, The Miracle of Gristle sidebar on page 18). Few things can devastate articular cartilage as quickly and as thoroughly as an intra-articular infection. The chemicals generated in the inflammatory response to infection are directly toxic to articular cartilage and can destroy it rapidly. For this reason, an infected joint is considered an orthopedic emergency.

▶ *Diagnosis*

In the absence of trauma, any hot, red, swollen joint should be considered infected until proven otherwise. Fever, elevated serum white cell count, elevated C-reactive protein, and an elevated erythrocyte sedimentation rate are all helpful, but not diagnostic. The best and most definitive test is a joint aspiration. Major joint arthrocentesis techniques are described in Chapter 9. If you suspect infection in a joint that you do not feel comfortable aspirating, then seek orthopedic consultation. Once the aspiration is completed, administer a single dose of broad-spectrum antibiotics and send the aspirate for the following studies:

1. **Aerobic and anaerobic culture and sensitivity.** It will take time for the cultures to yield results, but if it turns out that the joint is infected, these results will guide the choice of antibiotics.
2. **Gram stain.** If organisms are seen, the diagnosis of infection is confirmed. If no organisms are seen, infection may still be present (see discussion that follows).

fibers it innervates. For sensory nerve axons, the type of end organ will vary depending on the type of sensation the axon is conveying (pressure, temperature, pain, etc.). While it is controversial, there is some evidence that motor end plates and other end organs deteriorate in the absence of nerve stimulation. The longer the absence of stimulation is, the more likely it is that the end organ will deteriorate. If the end organ is gone by the time the healing axon reaches it, the healed nerve will not be able to serve its function. For this reason, distal nerve injuries have a better prognosis than proximal nerve injuries. This also explains why functional recovery from axonotmesis injuries is often less complete than it is with neuropraxia injuries.

The third, and most severe, type of nerve injury is called neurotmesis. In neurotmesis, the entire nerve, including the epineurium, is transected. Such nerve lacerations require end-to-end surgical repair if function is to be restored. Once the two ends of the transected nerve are sewn together, the healing process is identical to that seen with an axonotmesis injury. The axons degenerate distal to the injury, and the severed proximal ends of the axons grow down the vacant endoneurial conduits to reach their end organs. If the severed nerve is not repaired, then the sprouting axons grow out into the surrounding scar tissue, forming a disorganized ball of tangled, randomly oriented nerve endings called a neuroma. Although early repairs have a better prognosis than late repairs, 6 weeks after injury is still considered "early," and nerve repairs can be successful if they are initiated 3-6 months after the nerve has been transected.

If a transected nerve is discovered in the exploration of a traumatic wound, it is typically repaired expediently. In most cases of nerve dysfunction following closed orthopedic trauma, however, there is no open wound, and the integrity

(continued on following page)

of the nerve cannot be assessed visually. Electrodiagnostic studies will not show fibrillation potentials until about 6 weeks after injury, so electromyographic/nerve conduction study (EMG/NCS) evaluation does not aid in diagnosing the severity of nerve injury in the acute setting. Imaging studies such as MRI or ultrasound may not visualize the anatomy of the nerve well enough to detect a lacerated nerve in most cases.

So, in our example of a Colles fracture in which the patient's sensory exam does not normalize after correction of the fracture deformity, the only way to establish whether the nerve is severed is to make an incision and surgically explore the nerve at the site of the fracture. Statistically, by far the most common finding in such cases of immediate exploration is that the nerve is intact. In fact, it is so unlikely that the nerve will be severed that surgical exploration (which creates more trauma and further disrupts the blood supply to the injury site) is not recommended. Overwhelmingly, the odds are that the nerve injury is a neuropraxia or axonotmesis, in which case the nerve recovers on its own over time. EMGs can be used to detect fibrillation potentials at 6 weeks, and, in the rare cases in which improvement is not observed clinically or electrodiagnostically in 6-12 weeks, then surgical exploration is recommended to determine if the nerve was severed so that nerve repair can be undertaken.

So, if the sensory exam of a patient with a traumatic orthopedic deformity (fracture or dislocation) is abnormal, this is considered an emergency. It is considered an emergency because the nerve is so deformed that its function is altered, and the longer the nerve is left in this position, the more severe the nerve injury is likely to become. Neuropraxia injuries can become axonotmesis injuries, and the prognosis for complete recovery worsens. If the neurologic exam does not normalize after the deformity has

(continued on following page)

3. **Crystals.** The shape and appearance of joint fluid crystals under polarized light microscopy can aid in diagnosing gout (long, needle-shaped negatively birefringent monosodium urate crystals are typical of gout) and pseudogout (shorter, rhomboidal crystals that are positively birefringent under polarized light are typical of pseudogout).

4. **Cell count.** Joint fluid that has greater than 50,000 white blood cells per high-power field should be considered diagnostic for infection. Other inflammatory conditions, such as gout and pseudogout, will rarely result in a leukocytosis of this magnitude.

If the Gram stain and cell count are negative, discontinue antibiotics and await culture results. If the Gram stain shows organisms in the synovial fluid *or* the cell count of the synovial fluid has more than 50,000 white blood cells per high-power field, then timely surgical irrigation is recommended. A few of the organisms that cause intra-articular infections can be effectively treated with antibiotics alone and no surgery. The old (penicillin-sensitive) gonococcus was a great example. A few doses of antibiotics would successfully kill all of these bacteria in the joint. But, even in cases where the infection can be treated with antibiotics, surgical irrigation is recommended since dead bacteria in the joint still present antigens that elicit the violent inflammatory response that is so harmful to the articular surfaces.

To best protect the articular cartilage surfaces inside a joint, it is important to identify and treat intra-articular infections promptly. The consequences of articular surface damage are most severe in large, weight-bearing joints like the ankle, knee, and hip. Infections of the interphalangeal joints of the toes and fingers and joints like the acromioclavicular joint of the shoulder are often treated as urgent, but not emergent, conditions. If the articular cartilage of the joint is already badly damaged from another preexisting condition (osteoarthritis, for example) and the patient is not systemically ill from the infection, the infection can be considered less of an emergency. If the articular cartilage surfaces have been replaced with metal and plastic (as is the case with total knee, hip, and shoulder replacements), then the condition is urgent but not an emergency. Ultimately, the provider's judgment must play a role as we decide how aggressively to treat potential joint infections, and numerous clinical factors have to be considered.

OPEN FRACTURES

Fractures in which there is a laceration or soft tissue loss that permits communication between the external environment and the fracture site are called *open fractures*. These fractures are considered orthopedic emergencies because they put the patient at risk for bone infection (osteomyelitis), which can be chronic and debilitating. In severe cases of chronic osteomyelitis, the only way to eradicate the infection is to amputate the extremity. To serve its purpose of providing a structurally rigid framework onto which our muscles attach, cortical bone has to be dense and strong. It has very few voids in it for cells to occupy and very few channels in it to accommodate blood vessels because these features would weaken it. The resulting material is strong, but being relatively acellular and avascular, it is prone to infection, and once infection is established in bone, it is hard to eliminate. In an attempt to minimize the chances of an open fracture developing osteomyelitis, a standard treatment protocol has been adopted by most orthopedic practitioners.

1. **Start broad-spectrum intravenous antibiotics.**
2. **Debride the wound of any obvious gross contamination.**
3. **Apply an occlusive dressing.** Gauze and tape will suffice. The goal is to cover and protect the open wound.
4. **Splint the extremity.** This prevents motion at the fracture site from further injuring adjacent soft tissues. This can be a simple splint made of cardboard and tape if more sophisticated materials aren't available.
5. **Initiate formal irrigation and debridement in the operating room as soon as is practical.**

Factors such as the degree of contamination, the patient's medical health (diabetes and peripheral vascular disease are conditions that worsen the prognosis) and the amount of soft tissue damage all play a role in determining the urgency with which these injuries must be treated, but, in most cases, the consensus among orthopedists is that these injuries need to be treated as emergencies.

been corrected, then the condition is observed, and if improvement is not seen at 6 weeks, an EMG exam is administered. If, at the time of injury, treatment of the fracture involves a surgical dissection (e.g., the Colles fracture requires plate-and-screw fixation), then it is recommended that the malfunctioning nerve be explored during that procedure, but a surgical dissection for the sole sake of exploring the nerve is not indicated.

If the neurologic exam were normal before the fracture or dislocation was reduced and after the correction of the deformity the neurologic exam is found to change and become abnormal, then timely surgical exploration is indicated. In these cases, it is possible that the nerve is caught in the fracture site, and surgery is the only safe way to address this problem.

DISLOCATIONS

In the section on neurovascular injuries, we discussed dislocations because they can create deformities that can result in nerve or vascular compression. Dislocations without associated neurovascular compromise are also considered orthopedic emergencies. Figure 7-10 shows a glenohumeral joint dislocation of the shoulder. In injuries like this one, the ball is often "perched" on the edge of the socket. Contact pressures at the site of rim contact against the ball can permanently damage articular cartilage. Furthermore, the ball is pressed tight against the joint capsule, leaving no room for synovial fluid. Because articular cartilage has no intrinsic blood supply, it relies on passive diffusion of nutrients from the surrounding synovial fluid, and that phenomenon is greatly compromised when the joint is dislocated. Dislocations also subject the joint capsule and surrounding soft tissues to significant tension, which, over time, can damage these structures irreversibly and make achieving a stable relocation more difficult. Last, the increased periarticular

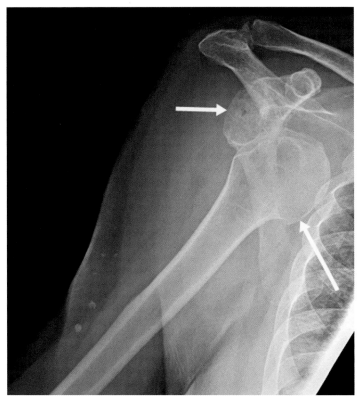

Figure 7-10. A dislocation of the glenohumeral joint of the shoulder. In general, this and other large joint dislocations are considered emergencies.

soft tissue tension can compromise blood flow to the joint. This can lead to avascular necrosis. Hip dislocations are especially prone to this problem (see the sidebar, Why Is the Femoral Head Prone to Avascular Necrosis? on page 98 in Chapter 3).

If you encounter a dislocated joint, perform and document a neurovascular exam, reduce the dislocation, or, if you don't feel comfortable doing so, call someone who can. After the joint is reduced, immobilize the extremity and reevaluate the neurovascular exam, then confirm that the joint has been successfully reduced with a postreduction x-ray.

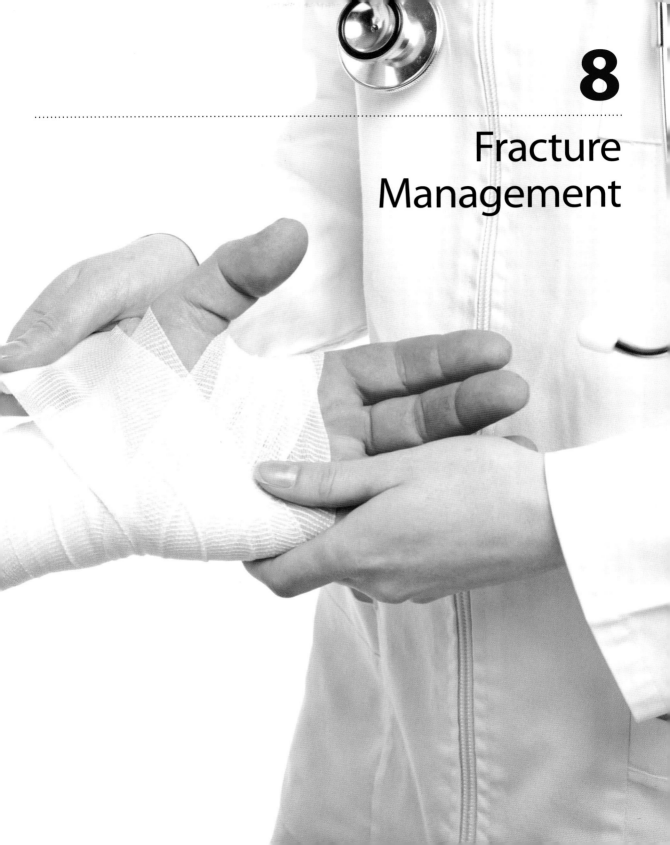

8

Fracture
Management

WHY TREAT FRACTURES?

What are the goals of fracture treatment? What do we aim to accomplish when we treat these injuries? The best way to answer these questions is to imagine what would happen if we left the fracture untreated. Without some form of stabilization, fractures can be excruciatingly painful, and pain control is front and center among the goals of fracture treatment. A splint, a cast, traction, or surgical fixation, all of these options for fracture treatment stabilize the injured skeleton and significantly reduce the pain associated with it. Treating the fracture also reduces the deformity. Most fractures result in some degree of deformity. Sometimes, the deformity is significant; sometimes it is not. If the deformity is significant, leaving it uncorrected would have negative consequences in terms of musculoskeletal function. Furthermore, deformed bones transmit abnormal

(continued on following page)

Fractures are relatively common orthopedic injuries, and anyone providing primary patient care is likely to encounter them. Although a complete and thorough treatment of this subject would require an entire textbook in and of itself, a chapter explaining the basic principles of fracture care seems appropriate for any textbook that covers office orthopedics.

NOMENCLATURE

There are a handful of terms used to describe fractures that are important to know and understand. These terms and their definitions are reviewed in the material that follows. Until the recent increase in our ability to share x-ray images using social media–based devices, the terms used to accurately describe fractures were critical. These terms helped orthopedic providers conjure up a mental picture of the fracture that was being described to them as they received consults over the phone. These days, providers can quickly and easily share x-rays on smartphones (patient-identifying information excluded, of course). As a result, the ability to accurately describe a fracture is becoming a lost art. When ordering x-rays, always order an anteroposterior (AP) and a lateral view (or two other orthogonal views). Figure 8-1 demonstrates how a broken bone can look perfectly aligned on one view (as the tibia looks on the AP view in Figure 8-1A) and be poorly aligned on the second view (see how angulated the tibia fracture is on the

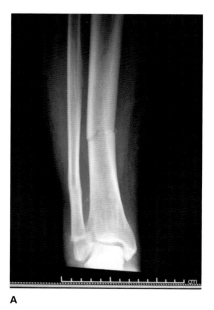
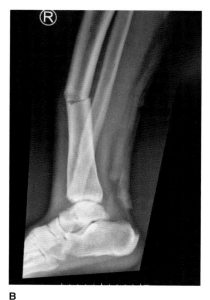

A   **B**

Figure 8-1. An AP (**A**), and lateral (**B**) x-ray of a tibia and fibula (tib-fib) fracture demonstrating how the fracture can appear well aligned on one view and displaced on the other. When getting x-rays to evaluate an injured extremity, it is important to obtain at least two views at 90 degrees (orthogonal) to each other.

lateral view in Figure 8-1B). The fracture of the distal tip of the fibula also appears to be reasonably well aligned on the AP view, but we can appreciate that it is 100% displaced on the lateral view. If a long bone (like the tibia, femur, or humerus) is being studied, AP and lateral x-rays should include the joints above and below the fracture. This may not be practical in all cases, but strictly speaking, that is the protocol.

In orthopedics, we use the term *fracture* to describe any injury that disrupts the structure of a bone. For instance, we would consider a tiny "hairline" crack a fracture, and an injury that breaks a bone into two unconnected pieces is also a fracture. Also, we don't use the term *compound fracture*. To some, a compound fracture is any severely displaced fracture. To others, the term indicates that the bone has penetrated through the skin. In orthopedics, we have other terms we use to describe these injuries, and we avoid using the term *compound fracture* because of the confusion it creates. The basic terms used in describing fractures are provided next.

Intra-articular/Extra-articular

The terms intra-articular and extra-articular are used to indicate whether the fracture we are describing enters into an adjacent joint. Figure 8-2 shows an intra-articular fracture of the proximal

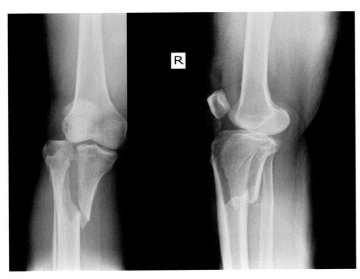

Figure 8-2. An intra-articular fracture of the proximal tibia (*Licensed from Shutterstock*).

tibia. The fracture enters the knee joint. The fracture in Figure 8-3 is an extra-articular fracture of the same bone. The fracture shown in Figure 8-3 does not enter the joint.

forces to the joints above and below them, which can cause premature wear of articular cartilage and early arthritis. A primary goal in the treatment of fractures with significant deformity is to correct the deformity so that these adverse consequences can be avoided. Also, it is usually the case that placing the fractured bone fragments in close apposition and then limiting the motion of the fracture increases the chances that the fracture will heal and achieve a bony union. When fractures don't heal with a solid bony union, we call them *nonunions*. When they heal, but heal in abnormal alignment, we call them *malunions*. So, the basic goals of fracture management are to decrease pain, correct deformity, and increase the chances of fracture healing.

One of the oldest treatments for fractured extremities is traction. If you throw a pearl necklace onto the floor, it can come to rest in about any shape or configuration you can imagine. But if you pull the two ends of that necklace in opposite directions, the necklace will automatically assume the shape of a straight line. That is the principle behind the use of traction to treat long-bone extremity fractures. Applying traction to the foot, for example, will pull an angulated fracture of the femur or tibia straight. For decades, extremity fractures, especially those in the tibia and femur, were treated in traction.

Successful fracture treatment requires that we accomplish two things: (1) put the fractured bone(s) in the proper position (a step orthopedists call *reducing* the fracture or *obtaining a reduction*) and (2) *maintain that reduction* until the fracture has healed. Traction is capable of accomplishing both goals, and it was used to do so with good results for a large part of the history of orthopedics. In the 1940s and 1950s, a big part of any orthopedist's job was to make hospital rounds on a legion of patients who were in the hospital in bed in skeletal traction waiting for their

(continued on following page)

fractures to heal. Hospitals were full of patients like the one shown in Figure 8-A.

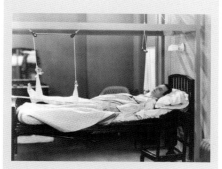

Figure 8-A. A patient in traction for a lower extremity fracture (*Licensed from Shutterstock*).

These fractures take a long time to heal, so a patient's length of stay was often between 1 and 3 *months*, an eternity by today's standards. With the long periods of bed rest that traction required came all of the attendant complications of immobility. Deep venous thrombosis, pulmonary emboli, pneumonia, pressure ulcers, the list goes on and on. These complications forced the evolution of orthopedics to focus on new treatments and procedures that would mobilize patients faster. For the most part, traction was replaced with open reduction/internal fixation operations, or ORIFs. In these procedures, the skin is *opened*, and the fracture is *reduced* back into its anatomic alignment. An *internal* means of *fixation* (a rod or a plate and screws) is employed to maintain the reduction until the bone has healed. One of the few examples of the use of traction in contemporary orthopedics is the external fixator. Figure 8-B shows an external fixator apparatus being used in the treatment of a distal radius fracture. Two metal pins are drilled through the skin and into the index finger metacarpal bone. A second set of two more pins is drilled through the skin and into the proximal radius. The two pairs

(continued on following page)

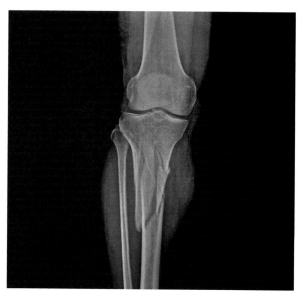

Figure 8-3. An extra-articular fracture of the proximal tibia (*Licensed from Shutterstock*).

Displaced/Nondisplaced

The terms displaced and nondisplaced help convey how far apart the broken pieces of bone (fracture fragments) are separated from each other or from their normal anatomic position. Technically speaking, *all* fractures are displaced *some* amount if we can see the fracture on an x-ray. The tiny radiolucent line that we see when we examine the x-ray of a bone with a hairline fracture is only there because the fracture fragments have separated (displaced) from one and other far enough to create a void, or gap. In living bone, that void is initially filled with blood. Because the density of blood is much less than the density of bone, blood does not block the x-ray beam as well as bone does, so the blood-filled gap appears on the x-ray as a radiolucent line. We generally consider fractures that are displaced a millimeter or two "nondisplaced," even though they *are* displaced a small amount. Fractures in which the fragments are separated by a centimeter or more in smaller bones, or several centimeters in larger bones, are described as "widely displaced." Other terms you will encounter that aim to describe fracture fragment displacement are "moderately displaced" and "minimally displaced." Obviously, all of this is rather subjective. If you are uncertain how to describe the displacement of a particular fracture, you can always quantitate the displacement in millimeters.

Figure 8-4 shows a fracture of the proximal ulna at the elbow joint. I would estimate that the fracture fragments in Figure 8-4 are displaced about 1 mm. We could either describe this fracture as "an extra-articular fracture of the proximal ulna that is minimally

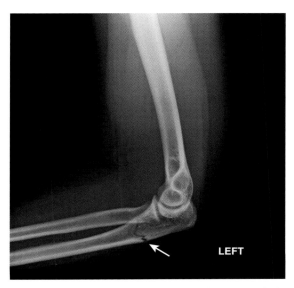

Figure 8-4. A minimally displaced (1 mm) fracture of the proximal ulna (see arrow) (*Licensed from Shutterstock*).

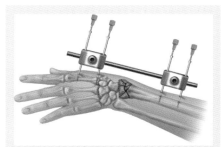

Figure 8-B. An external fixator.

of pins are connected with a rigid frame. The length of this frame can be adjusted to increase the distance between the two sets of pins, applying traction to the fracture. An external fixator is essentially a mobile form of local traction.

displaced" or "an extra-articular fracture of the proximal ulna that is 1 mm displaced." If you want to be precise, you can measure the displacement on the x-ray with a ruler, but an estimate will suffice. All that is really important is that we differentiate displaced fractures from those that are minimally or not displaced. Figure 8-5

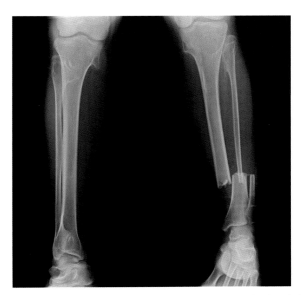

Figure 8-5. A widely displaced fracture of the distal tibia and fibula (tib-fib) (*Licensed from Shutterstock*).

CAN FRACTURES CAUSE ARTHRITIS?

The answer is yes, absolutely! In the ankle joint, for example, fractures are the leading cause of arthritis. There are four ways in which fractures lead to arthritis in the joints adjacent to them.

1. **Direct injury resulting in the death of the chondrocytes in articular cartilage.** If the bone is injured by a force large enough to break it, it is possible that that same force dealt a fatal blow to some of the cartilage cells on the articular surface. When these cells die, the cartilage deteriorates, resulting in post-traumatic arthritis.

2. **Long-bone fractures that heal with angular deformities subject adjacent joints to abnormal forces.** The femur shaft fracture shown in Figure 8-C healed with an angular deformity that affects the weight-bearing forces on the knee below it, shifting those forces

(continued on following page)

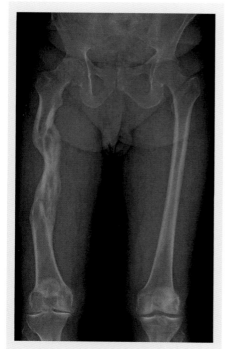

Figure 8-C. A malunion of the femur that alters the forces across the knee joint (*Licensed from Shutterstock*).

disproportionately toward the medial side of the joint. As a result, the medial articular cartilage of the knee joint will wear away faster, and the patient may develop bone-on-bone knee joint arthritis. The consequences of angular deformities in long bones are more serious in weight-bearing joints, where the forces are higher. A fracture of the humerus with angular deformity similar to that shown in Figure 8-C would be less likely to result in post-traumatic arthritis of the shoulder joint above or of the elbow joint below because the forces on these non–weight-bearing joints are much lower.

3. **Intra-articular fractures that disrupt the shape of the articular surface of a bone in a joint.** Figure 8-15 shows a tibial plateau fracture that has altered

(continued on following page)

shows a fracture that is widely displaced, and the femur fracture in Figure 8-6 is *extremely* displaced.

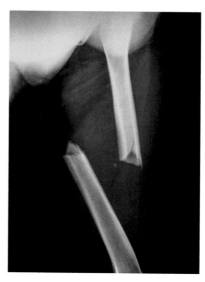

Figure 8-6. A fracture of the femur demonstrating extreme displacement (*Licensed from Shutterstock*).

Comminution

The term *comminution* refers to the number of bone fragments that result from a fracture. In general, we describe fractures with three or more fracture fragments as "comminuted," and those with more than four or five fracture fragments as "highly comminuted." Figure 8-6 shows a fracture in which the distal femur is broken into two, separate, widely displaced pieces (fragments). The fragments are widely displaced, but this is not a comminuted fracture. Figure 8-7 shows a highly comminuted fracture of the tibia with many different fracture lines and fragments.

Open/Closed

If there is communication between the fracture and the outside environment through a laceration or other defect in the skin, we consider the fracture to be an "open fracture." Open fractures are associated with a high risk of infection and require immediate evaluation by an orthopedist, emergency room physician, or other qualified provider.

Fracture-Dislocation

A fracture-dislocation is a fracture adjacent to a joint dislocation. Figure 8-8 shows a fracture-dislocation of the elbow. In this example, the ulna is broken, and the joint between the radius and

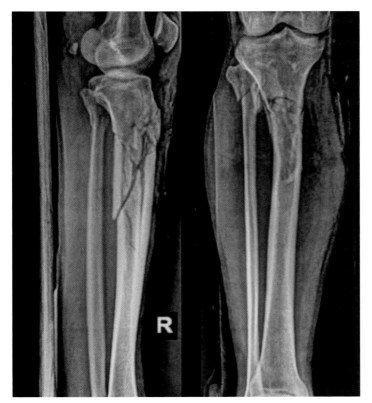

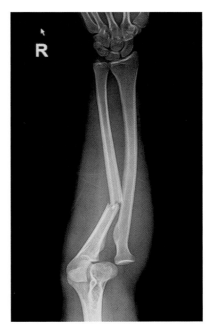

Figure 8-8. A fracture dislocation of the elbow. The radius is dislocated; the ulna is fractured (*Licensed from Shutterstock*).

Figure 8-7. A comminuted fracture of the proximal tibia (*Licensed from Shutterstock*).

the humerus is dislocated. Figure 8-9A shows a fracture dislocation of the ankle. When you compare it to the x-ray of a normal ankle (Figure 8-9B), you'll see that the posterior part of the distal tibia has broken (yellow arrow), allowing the talus bone to dislocate posteriorly (white arrow). The wrist injury in Figure 8-10 may appear at first glance to be a fracture-dislocation, but the wrist joint is not dislocated. The carpal bones are articulating properly with the end of the radius, but there is a widely displaced, extra-articular fracture of the radius.

Location

When describing fractures, it is helpful not only to identify which bone is broken, but also to make some attempt to identify *where* on the bone the fracture has occurred. Figure 8-11 shows the names given to the different parts of a typical bone. The long, tubular, center section is called the shaft, or the *diaphysis*. The parts of the bone toward the ends of the bone where the bone starts to flare out and widen are called the *metaphysis*, and the very ends of the bone are called the *epiphysis*. In the skeletally immature bones of

the shape of the proximal tibia significantly. Left uncorrected, this deformity will likely heal in this position, resulting in a loss of the normal congruity between the surface of the femur and the surface of the tibia in the joint. The resulting mismatch in the shapes of these bones will accelerate the wear rate of the articular cartilage and can lead to post-traumatic arthritis in the knee joint. The ankle and the knee are particularly susceptible to the post-traumatic arthritis caused by intra-articular fractures because they are weight-bearing joints, and they have a normal range of motion that is limited to a single flexion/extension plane. The hip joint is also a weight-bearing

(continued on following page)

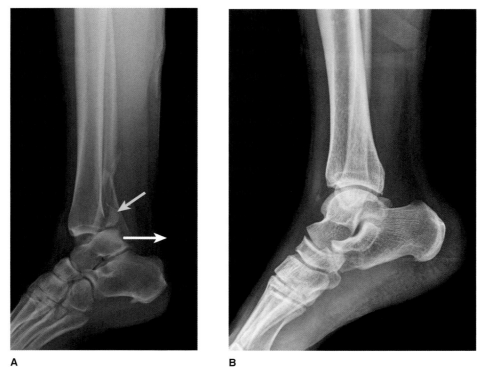

A　　　　　　　　　　　　　　　　　　**B**

Figure 8-9. A fracture dislocation of the ankle. The distal tibia is fractured, and the ankle (tibio-talar) joint is dislocated (*Images licensed from Shutterstock*).

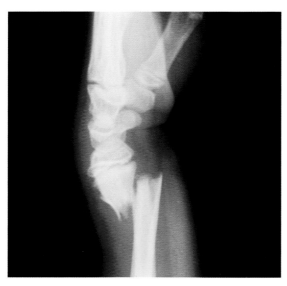

Figure 8-10. A widely displaced fracture of the distal radius. You might initially think that the wrist is dislocated, but it is not. The distal radius fragment and the carpal bones are articulating normally, but the hand, wrist, and distal radius fracture fragment are all displaced from the shaft of the radius (*Licensed from Shutterstock*).

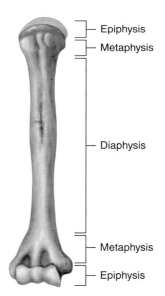

Epiphysis

Metaphysis

Diaphysis

Metaphysis

Epiphysis

Figure 8-11. The names given to the individual parts of a typical long bone.

children who have not yet finished growing, there is an uncalcified section in the bone between the metaphysis and the epiphysis that is the growth plate, or the *physis*. In very young bones, the entire epiphysis and parts of the metaphysis and diaphysis are not yet calcified and appear radiolucent on x-ray. Figure 8-12 shows an x-ray

joint, but it is a universal joint that can move in any plane of motion, allowing it to shift its position and better distribute abnormal forces over its articular surfaces.

4. **Fracture healing often increases the density of bone, decreasing its elasticity.** Figure 8-D shows a cross section of a typical bone

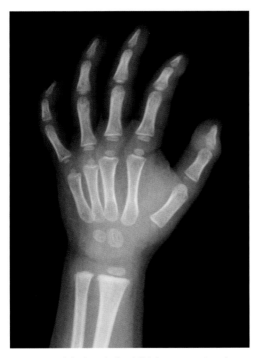

Figure 8-12. An x-ray of the hand of a child demonstrating that many of the bones in the skeleton at this age are made of uncalcified cartilage. These yet-to-be-calcified bones are not visible on an x-ray (*Licensed from Shutterstock*).

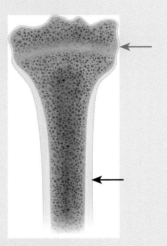

Figure 8-D. A drawing showing the bony architecture of the proximal end of the tibia. In the diaphysis (shaft) of the bone, the cross-sectional area is small and the cortical walls are thick. In the metaphysis and epiphysis, the cross-sectional area is large and the cortical walls are thin.

of the hand and wrist of an infant. Only the diaphysis of the ulna bone is calcified and is visible on the x-ray. The diaphysis and the center of the distal metaphysis of the radius are calcified and appear on the film. The epiphysis of the ulna and six of the eight carpal bones are there, but they are composed of cartilage, not bone, so we can't see them. As the child grows, the cartilage will calcify and become visible on x-ray. One of the challenges faced when caring for children with bony injuries is that fractures through the cartilaginous portions of the bone cannot be seen on x-ray.

The freshly calcified bone of a young skeleton is more flexible and softer than brittle adult bone, and it can deform in ways that adult bones cannot. Examples of fractures that are unique to pediatric bone include *greenstick fractures* (fractures in which the bone cracks or bends, but the two pieces of bone stay connected to one

(in this case, the tibia). The image also demonstrates an interesting aspect of the anatomy of our bones. Each bone has a hard, outer shell of dense *cortical bone* and a soft, inner matrix of porous *cancellous bone*. In the diaphysis (shaft) of bones like the tibia and femur, the layer of hard cortical bone is very thick. This thick, dense cortical bone is shown by the black arrow in Figure 8-D. At the proximal end of the tibia and the distal end of the femur,

(continued on following page)

the morphology of these bones starts to change. The dense cortical shell becomes paper thin (red arrow), and the bone flares out like the end of a trumpet. These expanded bone ends with relatively thin cortical walls and large volumes of softer, more elastic cancellous bone are thought to provide a shock-absorbing function that helps preserve the knee joint. Many bones are configured this way. Fractures that injure the wide, spongy sections of a bone heal with bone that is typically more dense and less elastic, making those bones less efficient shock absorbers.

another, like a green stick does when you try to snap it in half) and *torus,* or *buckle,* fractures (fractures in which the bone collapses like an accordion, but doesn't actually break). Figure 8-13 shows a typical greenstick fracture.

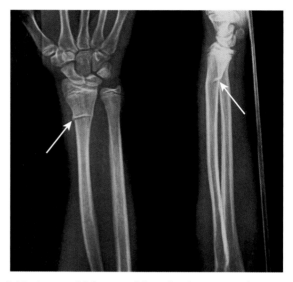

Figure 8-13. A greenstick fracture of the radius. In a greenstick fracture, part of the bone breaks and part of it bends (like a green stick) (*Licensed from Shutterstock*).

We will often try to describe the geometry of the fracture (oblique or transverse) and the type of deformity (angulated, shortened, and translated). Figure 8-5 shows a transverse, widely displaced fracture of the diaphysis of the distal third of the tibia that is translated laterally with minimal shortening. Figure 8-14 shows a long oblique fracture of the mid diaphysis of the femur with shortening and an angular deformity.

SPECIAL FRACTURE NAMES WORTH KNOWING

Certain often-seen fracture patterns have been given special names. For instance, the fracture in Figures 8-2 and 8-15 is known as a *tibial plateau fracture.* By definition, all tibial plateau fractures are fractures of the proximal tibial metaphysis and epiphysis, so we can omit the terms that describe the location of the fracture in Figure 8-15 and just call this fracture a "highly comminuted, widely displaced right tibial plateau fracture." There are hundreds of fractures that have been given special names in orthopedics, and listed next are the ones you are most likely to encounter.

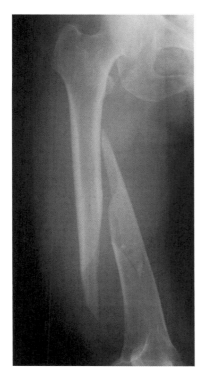

Figure 8-14. A long, oblique fracture of the shaft (diaphysis) of the femur that is displaced and angulated (*Licensed from Shutterstock*).

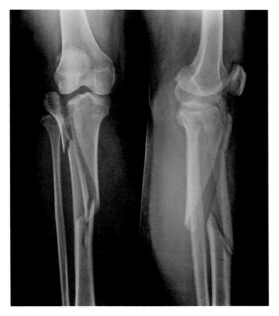

Figure 8-15. A tibial plateau fracture. This one is displaced, comminuted, and intra-articular (*Licensed from Shutterstock*).

Fracture: Special Name	Description
Boxer's Fracture 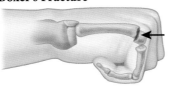	Fracture of the distal third of the fifth metacarpal
Colles Fracture 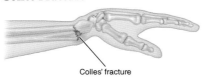 Colles' fracture	Fracture of the distal end of the radius with dorsal angulation or displacement
Jones Fracture 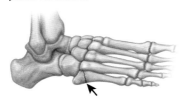	Fracture at the junction of the metaphysis and diaphysis of the proximal end of the fifth metatarsal
Dancer's Fracture 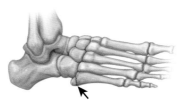	Fracture of the tuberosity (most proximal end) of the fifth metatarsal
Tibial Plateau Fracture 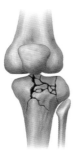	Fracture of the proximal end of the tibia, typically intra-articular

It is well beyond the scope of this book to try to delineate the treatment specifics for each and every specific fracture, but there are some basic principles worth understanding. With few exceptions, until they are healed, fractures that are not displaced simply need to be protected from the forces that could cause them to displace. Splints are usually used initially. Splints are a type of bandage that includes one or more rigid supports to immobilize the fracture. The safest and most conservative splint spans the joint above and below the fracture site. For instance, a radius fracture in the forearm would be treated with a splint that immobilizes the wrist joint distal to the fracture and the elbow joint proximal to the fracture. A tibia fracture would be treated with a splint that immobilizes the ankle joint below the fracture and the knee joint above. We often abbreviate the splints used for wrist fractures and omit the elbow, and very distal tibia fractures can often be treated with splints that do not include the knee, but, if you are not certain about how long a splint should be, the safest thing to do is to immobilize the joints above and below the fracture.

Splints do not need to be complicated and sophisticated to do their job. If nothing else is available, one can use a magazine and tape or cloth (Figure 8-16) to temporarily splint a wrist fracture

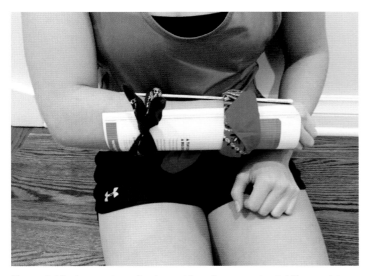

Figure 8-16. A magazine splint is a quick-and-easy way to stabilize a wrist injury.

while more definitive treatment is pursued. Be aware that all splints apply pressure to the skin, and that, over time, they can cause pressure ulcers. A splint that is going to be used for any significant amount of time needs to be well padded, and the patient needs to be instructed to report signs like loss of sensation, extreme swelling, and skin color changes, which could indicate that the splint is compromising the circulation of the extremity and may need to be loosened. In the initial hours to days after a fracture, splints are often preferred over casts because they allow for swelling.

Once the swelling decreases, we typically convert splints to casts. A cast is a circumferential rigid dressing that is more effective than a splint for immobilizing the fracture but can't expand to accommodate swelling. For most nondisplaced fractures, a cast is the definitive treatment. Casts are effective at protecting fractures from deforming forces, but the fracture should be monitored with x-rays throughout the healing process to ensure that it has not displaced. The frequency of x-ray monitoring will vary from fracture to fracture, but a safe approach would be to obtain an x-ray at 1 week, 3 weeks, and 6 weeks after initial cast application. Most healing fractures also have to be protected from the forces of weight bearing, which may require crutches, a walker, or even a wheelchair in some cases. Typical fracture-healing time is between 6 and 12 weeks.

Displaced fractures may need to be reduced and then immobilized with a cast or even an internal fixation operation. Be sure to review the section on open fractures and fractures with neurovascular compromise in Chapter 7. These are orthopedic emergencies and require expedient care.

SPECIAL CASES: FRACTURES THAT REQUIRE LESS ATTENTION

Next are listed a few fractures that can be treated more liberally than most, requiring less immobilization, shorter periods of protected weight bearing, or shorter healing times.

Rib Fractures

Rib fractures have an excellent blood supply and heal without any casting, splinting, or immobilization. An x-ray can be helpful in ruling out an associated pneumothorax, but the likelihood of a low-energy rib fracture, the type you would typically see in an outpatient setting, creating a pneumothorax is exceedingly small. A pneumothorax is usually associated with high-energy chest trauma.

Clavicle Fractures

Unless the fracture fragments are threatening to protrude through the skin, clavicle fractures (Figure 8-17) can all be treated conservatively. There are some data to support surgical treatment of widely displaced clavicle fractures, but this remains somewhat controversial. Like the ribs, the clavicle receives an excellent blood supply, and the vast majority of these fractures heal no matter how they are treated. A sling works just as well as a figure-of-eight brace or any other immobilization device, and the patient can come out

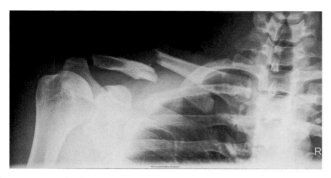

Figure 8-17. A displaced, transverse, and midshaft clavicle fracture (*Licensed from Shutterstock*).

of the sling as soon as comfort permits. A typical treatment plan for almost any clavicle fracture would be 4 weeks in a sling, followed by 4-6 weeks out of the sling, during which time motion is encouraged, but the patient is advised not to lift anything heavier than a cup of coffee. If x-rays at this time show that the fracture is healed, weight training may be initiated at 3 months. No contact sports should be undertaken until x-rays show that the fracture has healed and 3-6 months have passed since the injury.

Radial Head/Neck Fractures

The radial head/neck fractures of the proximal end of the radius at the elbow are common (Figure 8-18). They are unique because

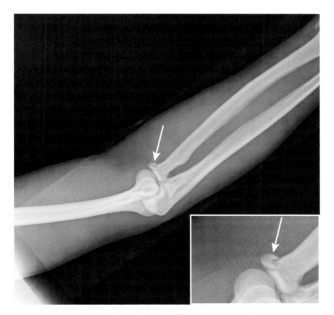

Figure 8-18. A fracture of the radial head (arrow) (*Licensed from Shutterstock*).

most of them don't require surgery *or* any form of immobilization. They are typically stable, meaning their displacement is unlikely to increase during the time it takes for them to heal. Only those rare fractures with large, widely displaced fragments of the radial head or the few examples that are associated with elbow joint instability require surgery, and while a splint may be used for 7-10 days for patient comfort, it is best *not* to immobilize these fractures. Because they create bleeding inside the elbow joint and that blood can mature into scar tissue, it is best to avoid immobilization and start moving the elbow joint as soon as possible to avoid stiffness.

Toe Fractures

While some would argue that certain displaced, intra-articular fractures of the big toe might require surgery, fractures in the bones of the lesser toes can be treated nonoperatively in almost every case (Figure 8-19). If the fracture creates a grotesque deformity of the

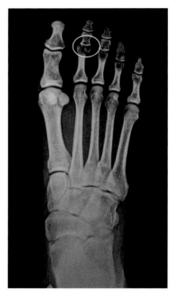

Figure 8-19. A comminuted, displaced, and intra-articular fracture of the distal end of the proximal phalanx of the second toe (*Licensed from Shutterstock*).

toe, a closed reduction and pinning may be recommended, but such toe fractures are rare. The garden-variety toe fracture creates pain, swelling, and bruising, but as long as the toe remains relatively straight (no matter how bad the x-ray looks), no surgery, splint, or cast is needed. The broken toe can be buddy taped to an adjacent toe, and, in severe cases, a special shoe with a rigid, inflexible sole can be used for a few weeks. Such shoes help control the pain of a toe fracture by limiting how much the toe moves when the patient walks.

Proximal Humerus Fractures

The shoulder joint is a unique joint in that it is truly a universal joint (Figure 8-20). Unlike a hinge joint like the knee, which only

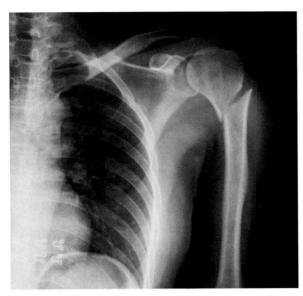

Figure 8-20. A moderately displaced, extra-articular fracture of the proximal metaphysis of the humerus (*Licensed from Shutterstock*).

moves in one plane of motion, it can move in almost any direction. This gives it a unique capacity to compensate for small rotational or angular deformities that result from proximal humerus fractures. Only proximal humerus fractures that disrupt the integrity of the articular surface or are very widely displaced require surgery. The rest can be treated in a sling for 2-3 weeks for comfort, then started on a physical therapy program that typically progresses from passive motion to active motion to progressive resistance exercises (weight lifting) over the course of 8-12 weeks.

Pubic Ramus Fractures

The superior and inferior pubic rami of the pelvis are non–weight-bearing parts of the skeleton (Figure 8-21). They offer important attachment points for major muscle groups, but our body weight is not supported by these bones. As a result, patients with superior or inferior pubic ramus fractures are allowed full weight bearing as soon as pain permits. These fractures do not require surgery, no matter how bad they may appear on x-ray, and there is no practical way to immobilize them with a cast or a splint. They typically occur in older patients for whom prolonged bed rest is associated

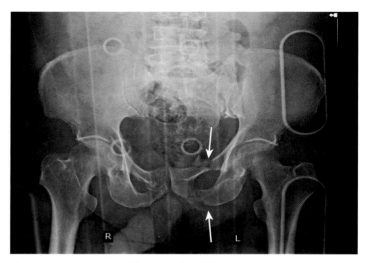

Figure 8-21. Comminuted fractures of the left superior and inferior pubic rami (arrows) (*Licensed from Shutterstock*).

with significant complications, so the prescription for these injuries is physical therapy with an emphasis on early mobilization and weight bearing as tolerated.

SPECIAL CASES: FRACTURES THAT REQUIRE MORE ATTENTION

If you read the sidebar in Chapter 1 called The Miracle of Gristle (page 18), you will appreciate the importance of articular cartilage. This slick, slippery, numb bearing surface material coats the ends of our bones and serves as the articulating surface in our joints. It is amazing material, but it lacks the ability to heal or regenerate, and one of the challenges we all face as we go through life is trying to make it last as long as possible. When it wears away and exposes the raw bone beneath it, that raw bone, which is rough, abrasive, and richly innervated (not slick, slippery, and numb, like articular cartilage), becomes the bearing surface of the joint, and it is a poor bearing surface. The process of wearing the articular cartilage down to bone is called arthritis, and arthritic joints with exposed bone as their bearing surfaces are stiff and painful.

The type of fracture that is most notorious for putting patients at risk for post-traumatic arthritis is the *intra-articular* fracture, in which the fracture changes the shape of the articulating surface of the bone that is broken. If that shape change is left uncorrected, the bone will heal in that position, and its shape will no longer match the shape of the bone in the joint against which it is meant to articulate. This loss of joint congruity is like having a square peg in a round hole, and the mismatch accelerates how fast the joint wears out. The ankle joint, the knee joint, and the wrist joint are particularly sensitive to post-traumatic changes in surface congruity, so we try hard to protect nondisplaced intra-articular fractures in these joints from displacing, and we are aggressive about correcting deformities that alter the joint surfaces in them as well. An operation is often required to "put the puzzle pieces back together" and then to hold them in place with plates, screws, and other hardware to ensure that they heal in an anatomic position.

Another type of fracture that requires special attention is a fracture that injures a bone with poor blood supply. The "poster child" for this type of fracture is a fracture of the distal half of the diaphysis (shaft) of the tibia (Figure 8-22). The blood supply is the

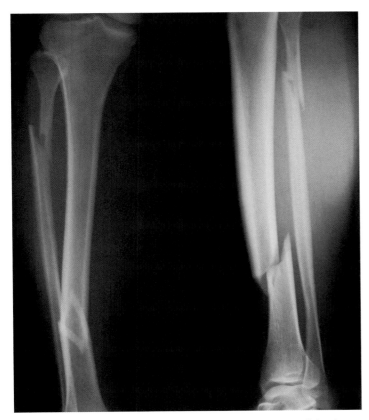

Figure 8-22. An oblique fracture at the junction of the middle and distal thirds of the tibia (*Licensed from Shutterstock*).

worst at the junction between the middle and distal thirds of this bone, and fractures in this area are prone to nonunion. Obtaining a satisfactory reduction, achieving adequate immobilization, and protecting the fracture with a period of non–weight-bearing all contribute to improving the odds of bony union. A history of smoking, venous stasis disease, atherosclerosis, and malnutrition all increase the chances of a poor result.

Another bone with a relatively inadequate blood supply is the scaphoid bone of the wrist (also known as the *carpal navicular* bone). Scaphoid fractures are common, and nondisplaced fractures can be hard to see on x-ray (Figure 8-23). Because the blood

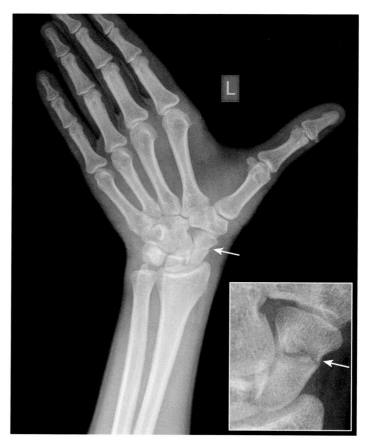

Figure 8-23. A scaphoid fracture (arrow) (*Licensed from Shutterstock*).

supply to the scaphoid bone is poor, these fractures take a long time to heal, and during that time, if not immobilized, nondisplaced fractures can displace, creating a deformity that predisposes the wrist to post-traumatic arthritis. Because initial x-ray changes can be subtle, it is recommended that any patient with a wrist injury who has tenderness over the anatomic snuffbox (a point on the wrist directly over the scaphoid bone; see Chapter 4 for details) be treated with a splint or cast that immobilizes the wrist and thumb and that x-rays be repeated 7-10 days after injury.

Local resorption of bone that occurs at the fracture site in the first week after injury makes the fracture easier to detect on the second set of x-rays. If a nondisplaced scaphoid fracture is diagnosed, treatment is 6-8 weeks in a cast that immobilizes the wrist and thumb (a thumb spica cast). Displaced fractures should be treated surgically to decrease the chances of post-traumatic arthritis.

As discussed in Chapter 3, the head of the femur has a notoriously poor blood supply. The few vessels that do nourish the femoral head reside in the femoral neck. If a patient sustains a displaced femoral neck fracture (Figure 8-24), these blood vessels

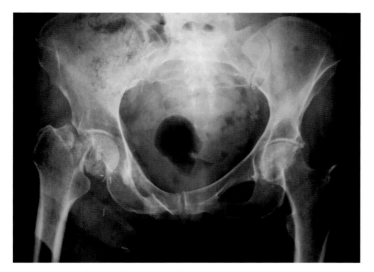

Figure 8-24. A displaced femoral neck fracture.

are interrupted and the femoral head is at risk for avascular necrosis. In older patients, displaced femoral neck fractures are treated with hip replacements because the risk of avascular necrosis is so high. A hip replacement is a poor choice for patients under 40 years of age. In this age group, the device will wear out and have to be revised multiple times; ultimately, the patient can have so many revisions that there can be no more revisions. For that reason, displaced femoral neck fractures in young patients are treated with immediate reduction and surgical fixation. Most of the data indicate that the shorter the period of time between the injury and surgical treatment, the better the chances are of avoiding avascular necrosis.

Spine Fractures

With the exception of atraumatic vertebral body compression fractures, fractures of the cervical, thoracic, and lumbar spine have to be regarded as potential emergencies. If these fractures displace, permanent injury to the spinal cord or spinal nerve roots can occur, and the consequences can be devastating. It is probably best that patients with these injuries be immobilized and transferred to an emergency department for imaging and evaluation.

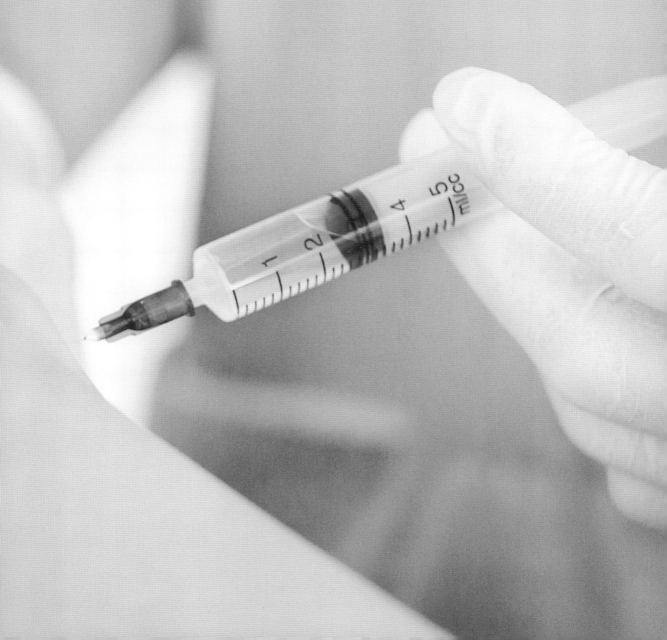

9

Injection Techniques

CORTICOSTEROIDS

If you are not using cortisone injections as a part of your treatment strategy for common orthopedic conditions, I strongly urge you to start. Corticosteroid injections are a safe and effective treatment option for many orthopedic diagnoses. They are inexpensive, easy to administer, and often provide quick and long-lasting relief of the pain associated with arthritis, tendonitis, bursitis, and many other conditions. These injections are extremely useful tools that any practitioner caring for ailments of the musculoskeletal system ought to know and use.

▶ *Frequency*

It is generally accepted that cortisone injections should be used judiciously. The specifics on this are somewhat vague. Some claim that the maximum frequency of injections for any one joint is one a month, not to exceed three per year. Others interpret the rule to be no more than one cortisone injection in any given joint every 4 months. The medical evidence supporting these guidelines remains elusive, but it is generally accepted that, given too frequently, cortisone can weaken connective tissue, including articular cartilage, tendons, and ligaments. What is even less clear is how many injections total a person can have (in any particular joint) in their lifetime. Some feel that patients should be limited to three injections (lifetime total) in any one joint. Others feel there is no lifetime limit, provided the rule of "one every 4 months" is not broken. Until a consensus can be reached, or until adequate medical evidence is put forth, it is certainly reasonable to inject any given joint with a maximum frequency of one injection every 4 months for a maximum duration of 3 years.

▶ *Sterile Technique*

Proper sterile technique is important. The inside of a joint or tendon sheath is similar to an abscess cavity. It is a dead space with relatively poor circulation. Infections grow easily in such spaces, and cortisone is known to have a weakening effect on the immune system, so there is a higher risk of creating an infection with an intra-articular corticosteroid injection than, say, an intramuscular injection such as an immunization. That said, the risk of infection from in-office cortisone injections is surprisingly low, on the order of 1 in 15,000. The practitioner need not wear sterile gloves, although a pair of unsterile gloves is recommended because there is a risk that the practitioner will come in contact with the patient's body fluids.

Prep an area of skin at the proposed injection site with betadine or chlorhexidine, then lay an alcohol square over the site where you plan to inject. The alcohol square is important because you can press on it with your fingertip and confirm that you are in the right spot without actually touching the sterile patch of skin where the needle will enter. When you are ready to inject, slide the alcohol square out of the way and proceed to pass the needle through the skin. Be sure not to touch and contaminate the needle as it passes into the target tissue.

▶ Systemic Effects

Very little of the injected corticosteroid is absorbed systemically, but, certainly, some very small amount is. Diabetics may report a transient (1- to 2-day) increase in blood sugar levels, and a few patients will experience facial flushing, increased heart rate, and dysphoria. These reactions are usually fairly mild and can be treated with an antihistamine such as Benadryl. Rarely, patients will report intense burning or aching pain at the injection site. This reaction, called a "steroid flare," is typically short lived (1-2 days) but can be severe enough to warrant the temporary use of narcotic pain relievers.

▶ Patients on Anticoagulation Therapy

All of the injection techniques reviewed here *except* the technique for administering a lumbar epidural steroid injection are safe to use on patients receiving systemic anticoagulation therapy. Remember that patients on warfarin therapy, for instance, routinely have their international normalized ratio (INR) measured by venipuncture. If they don't have bleeding complications from having a needle stuck directly and purposefully into a major vein, they are unlikely to have bleeding complications from one of these injections.

▶ Equipment and Materials

All injections should be prepared by someone who understands and practices good sterile technique. Handling the syringes, needles, and vials of medication has to be done with caution to avoid contamination. To prepare the skin, you will need a chemical skin prep (e.g., betadine or chlorhexidine), nonsterile gloves, and an alcohol square (see previous discussion). The injection will be a combination of corticosteroid and lidocaine *drawn up into the same syringe,* so that the patient can receive both medications with only one needle puncture. The preferred ratios of lidocaine and corticosteroid will vary from joint to joint and from practitioner to practitioner, but a typical large-joint (knee, shoulder, hip) injection would contain 1 mL (40 mg) of steroid and 4 mL of lidocaine. A typical medium-size joint (wrist, elbow, ankle, heel) injection would contain 1 mL of corticosteroid and 1 mL of lidocaine, and a small-joint injection (interphalangeal joints of toes or fingers) might typically contain ½ mL (20 mg) of corticosteroid and ½ mL of lidocaine. Most orthopedic offices prefer lidocaine *without* epinephrine. Although it is controversial, there is some evidence that epinephrine is a strong enough vasoconstrictor that it can cause ischemic damage when injected into small body parts like fingers and toes. Because many orthopedic offices treat hands and feet, lidocaine with epinephrine is not used to avoid inadvertently administering it into one of these areas.

The most commonly used corticosteroids are Kenalog and Depo-Medrol; both are equally effective. The desired concentration is 40 mg/mL. Be sure to choose a corticosteroid that is *in suspension*, not *in solution*. The difference is apparent on visual inspection of the medication in the glass vial in which it is packaged. Corticosteroids that are in solution are as clear as water. Those in suspension separate out into a watery liquid and a chalky, white powder that settles to the bottom of the vial until shaken, after which the medication appears milky white. The clear, watery-appearing preparations where the corticosteroid is in an aqueous solution should not be used for these injections. These medications are intended for situations where systemic administration is desired. For orthopedic injections, our goal is local, not systemic, treatment. Corticosteroid preparations that are in suspension are less apt to leave the joint or tendon sheath into which they are injected, although even with these preparations, a trace amount of the steroid can reach the systemic circulation. This is evidenced by the observation that diabetics who receive these injections will occasionally experience a transient increase in serum glucose levels (see previous discussion).

The best syringe to use is one with a Luer-Lock tip. Needles screw into the tip of the Luer-Lock syringe, making it harder for them to accidentally come off the tip of the syringe. If the syringe loaded with the injection to be used is stored vertically, with the needle end down (e.g., in the breast pocket of your white jacket), the chalky white powder can settle down into the hub of the needle and clog it. Even after vigorous shaking, the needle hub can be blocked enough that, when the plunger on the syringe is depressed, the needle pops off and the cortisone and lidocaine spray all over everything. This is always embarrassing (and it is universally agreed that such topical applications are far less effective!).

Needle choice is also important. A 1½-inch, 22-gauge needle will work well for almost every type of injection. The 1½ inches of needle length will get you into the knees and shoulders of all but the heaviest patients. An 18-gauge needle would be the ideal bore *from the standpoint of the injector.* One of the ways we determine that the needle is in the joint is to feel for the loss of resistance that occurs when the needle is in a free space like the inside of a joint or the subacromial space of the shoulder. Imagine your goal was to advance a needle through the wall of your cheek and into the inside of your mouth. If you are not deep enough, and the tip of the needle is still in the thick, dense tissue that makes up the wall of your cheek, you would encounter a lot of resistance as you attempt to push the plunger on the syringe. If the needle has successfully entered the empty space that is the inside of your mouth, then there is little resistance, and the plunger can be depressed easily. The presence or absence of resistance is important feedback that helps us know if our needle is where we want it to be, and those changes in resistance are easier to detect with a large-bore needle.

Our patients would prefer we use a 27-gauge needle. It hurts less. A 22-gauge needle is a good compromise. Its caliber is big enough that we can feel changes in resistance, but it is small enough in diameter not to hurt very much.

▶ *Anesthetizing the Skin*

Some practitioners will inject 1-2 mL of lidocaine or other local anesthetic with a small-gauge needle into the surface of the skin to anesthetize the area through which the needle will pass during the injection. This is certainly a reasonable thing to do. Another way to anesthetize the skin is to spray it with ethyl chloride. Ethyl chloride is liquid that evaporates quickly at room temperature, cooling the skin and making it less sensitive. It only works for a second or two after it is applied, so you have to work quickly. Once you have mastered an injection technique, you may find that it is easier for you and the patient to proceed without anesthetizing the skin. Most orthopedic injections are not particularly painful and can be done safely and effectively without this additional step.

▶ *Results*

Patients may experience immediate results during the lidocaine phase of the injection, but the anti-inflammatory effect of the corticosteroid can take several days to occur. Exactly when patients feel relief varies quite a bit from patient to patient. For practical reasons, I advise my patients that it can take up to 10 days to get the full effect (it takes my office 10 days to transcribe my office note and get it in the chart, so if they call me after 10 days to complain that they didn't get relief from the injection, I'll have my note for reference when we discuss alternative treatment options).

▶ *Final Tip*

If you're going to try skiing for the first time ever, don't go down a double black diamond, advanced, "experts-only" run. When trying any of these techniques for the first time, pick a thin, cooperative patient who will remain relaxed and tolerates needles well. If you are new to giving these injections, start with the easy ones like the hip greater trochanteric bursa or the lateral epicondyle of the elbow. For each of the injection techniques described in the following material, I have listed a "degree-of-difficulty" rating from 1 to 10, with 1 being the easiest and 10 being the hardest. I recommend starting with the simple ones and introducing the more difficult ones after you have built up your confidence and skill. Also, realize that many of the techniques described here involve touching bone with the tip of the needle. Fear not! This does not injure the patient.

KNEE: Intra-Articular Injection Technique

- **1 mL (40 mg) corticosteroid (Kenalog or Depo-Medrol); 4 mL lidocaine; 22-gauge, 1½-inch needle**
- **Patient position: supine on exam table**
- **Degree of difficulty: 3**

There are many different ways to successfully deliver an injection into the knee joint. The technique described here uses a superior-lateral approach. It is safe, easy, and effective. The patient is positioned supine with their knees relaxed and extended (Figure 9-1).

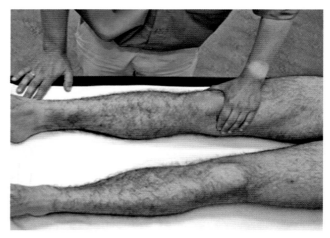

Figure 9-1. A patient lying supine on the exam table. This is the preferred position for the knee joint cortisone injection technique described here.

One advantage of this technique is that it is difficult for a patient in this position to watch the procedure. For some patients, watching the procedure can make them nervous and upset, and that makes it more difficult for them to relax. Also, in the rare case of a vaso-vagal event, the patient is safer in the supine position than in other positions, such as the seated position used for some knee injection techniques. You may need to rotate the patient's leg so that the patella is truly anterior because most patients will lie in slight external rotation when relaxed (Figure 9-2).

Prior to prepping the skin, the knee is palpated, and the proposed site is chosen. Try to feel the medial, lateral, superior, and inferior edges of the patella. If you are planning to inject with your right hand, place the index finger of your *left* hand on the medial edge of the patella and use the left hand to push the patella laterally. Our entry point is just posterior to the lateral edge of the superior half of the patella (Figure 9-3). Pushing the patella laterally makes

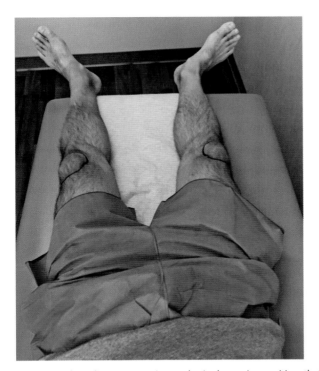

Figure 9-2. Note that when many patients relax in the supine position, their legs fall into an externally rotated position, and their patellae (circled) are no longer anterior, but rotated onto the lateral surface of the knee. To position the patella back onto the anterior surface of the knee, internally rotate the patient's legs.

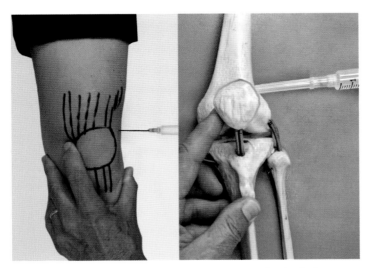

Figure 9-3. Preparing to give a knee joint injection. Use the tip of a finger on your other hand to push the patella laterally. This will make it easier to find the lateral edge.

it easier to identify the lateral edge of the patella, which is where the injection will be given. It is easier to get into the joint from the lateral side because the lateral quadriceps muscle doesn't come down as far (distally) as the medial quadriceps muscle does (Figure 9-4).

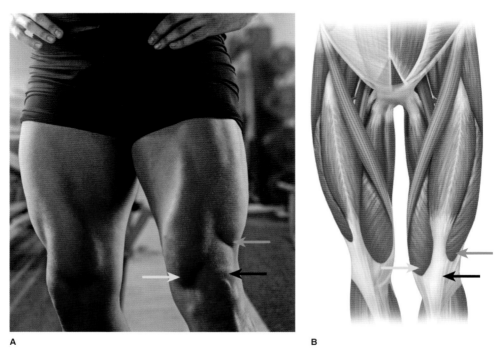

A   **B**

Figure 9-4. This photograph (**A**) and anatomic drawing (**B**) illustrate the fact that the medial quadriceps muscle inserts lower (yellow arrow) than the lateral quadriceps muscle (blue arrow). For this reason, we have to pass through less tissue if we chose to inject from the lateral side (black arrow) (*Image in* **A** *licensed from Shutterstock*).

On the lateral side of the patella, there is much less tissue between the surface of the skin and the inside of the knee joint, making it easier to get in from this direction.

It is helpful to imagine that the patella is a hockey puck resting on the top of a log. In this injection technique, our goal is to slide the needle under the puck. If we have positioned the patient properly, with the patella centered anteriorly, the flat undersurface of the patella is parallel to the ground, and our needle should be oriented parallel to the ground as well. If you look at a lateral view of the knee (Figure 9-5), you can see that the undersurface of the patella is not as flat as a hockey puck, it is shaped more like a rocker bottom that curves from superior to inferior. The patella is closest to the femur at its center point (black arrows in Figure 9-5), and because the space between the patella and femur is so tight there, that is a difficult place to try to enter the joint. The patella and femur diverge away from each other as you go above or below this center point, creating a bigger space for the needle. The space below the center point is occupied by the retropatellar fat pad, so it is best to aim for the space above (superior to) the center point (the space marked with a target in Figure 9-5).

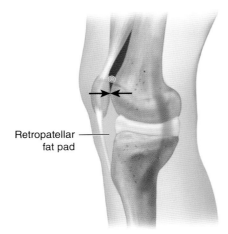

Figure 9-5. A drawing of a lateral view of the knee joint demonstrating that the tightest space between the patella and femur is actually in the very center (black arrows), and if you aim for a point just superior to this (target), the space is more open.

So, as you are preparing to give the injection and you are feeling the knee to better understand the location of the patella, identify the "equator" (the centerline that divides the patella into superior and inferior halves) of the patella and pick a point along the lateral edge of the patella that is about 2 centimeters above this centerline. The needle should enter the skin at this point, staying parallel to the ground and directed straight across toward the medial side as you advance into the joint (Figure 9-6).

Although we often refer to the different "compartments" of the knee joint (the medial compartment, the lateral compartment, the patella-femoral compartment), there are no true separate compartments. The inside of the knee is like the inside of your mouth. It is one big, open space, and anything injected into one compartment quickly flows into all of the other compartments. Technically, in the knee injection technique described here, the needle is entering the *patella-femoral* compartment, but because this compartment freely communicates with all of the rest of the knee joint, an injection given here delivers medication equally to the entire knee joint space.

It is important that the needle be advanced deep enough to pass completely through the skin and subcutaneous tissue and then

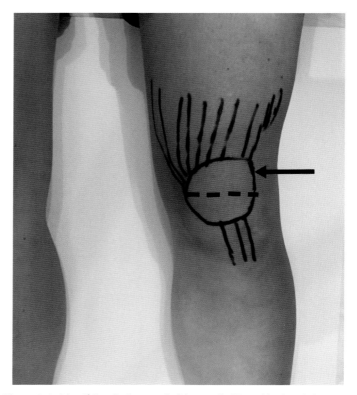

Figure 9-6. Identifying the "equator" of the patella (dotted line) and choosing an injection site about 2 centimeters superior to it (black arrow). Keep the needle parallel to the ground and directed straight across toward the medial side.

through the joint capsule to slide under the patella. Continuing the analogy between the knee and the mouth, to push a needle through your cheek and into the open space within your mouth, you have to make sure the needle makes it all the way through the "wall" of your cheek and into the open space inside your mouth. I recommend advancing the needle a full inch. If our desired target is a point deep to the upper third of the center of the patella, we will need to advance the needle at least an inch to get there (Figure 9-7). If you think your needle is in the proper place, but when you start to inject, there is a lot of resistance as you depress the plunger on the syringe, you may still be in the "cheek" of the knee, and you should advance the needle in deeper. If the needle is in the right spot, there should be little resistance as you inject. Remember to keep the index finger of your other hand pushing on the medial side of the patella. If you insert the needle and feel it contact bone, resist the temptation to pull the needle back. Leave the needle touching the bone and give the patella a couple quick shoves with your index finger. If the needle moves, your needle is on the patella and you need to try again with a more *posterior* entry point. If the

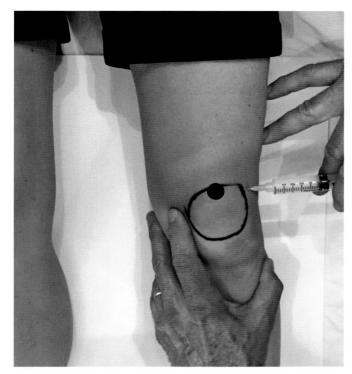

Figure 9-7. The black dot marks how far the needle will need to go to reach the center of the knee joint.

needle doesn't move, then the bone you are on is the femur and you need to try again using a more *anterior* entry point.

KNEE: Pes Tendon/Bursa Injection

- **1 mL (40 mg) corticosteroid (Kenalog or Depo-Medrol); 1 mL lidocaine; 22-gauge, 1½-inch needle**
- **Patient position: supine on exam table**
- **Degree of difficulty: 1**

The pes anserine (Latin for "goose foot") tendons are the tendons of the semitendinosus, sartorius, and gracilis muscles. They attach to the medial tibia a few centimeters inferior to the medial joint line of the knee in a pattern that resembles the three toes of the foot of a goose (Figure 9-8). If a patient has tenderness to palpation here, they may have a pes anserine tendonitis or bursitis. A cortisone injection can be a quick-and-easy remedy for this condition. Prep the skin over the point of maximal tenderness, then advance the needle until you feel it contact the surface of the tibia bone. The injection site is 3-4 centimeters distal to the medial joint line on the flat, subcutaneous surface of the tibia (Figure 9-9). Inject directly onto the surface of the tibia.

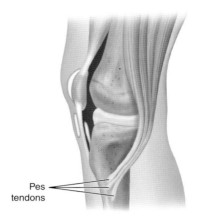

Figure 9-8. The tendons of the semitendinosus, sartorius, and gracilis muscles insert onto the anterior-medial tibia in a pattern that resembles a goose's foot.

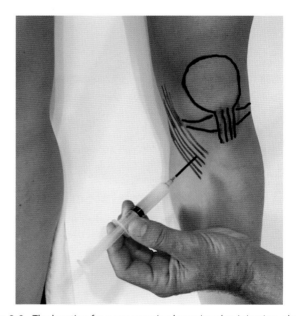

Figure 9-9. The location for a pes anserine bursa/tendon injection, about 2-3 centimeters distal to the joint line on the anterior-medial tibia.

SHOULDER: Subacromial Space Injection

- 1 mL (40 mg) corticosteroid (Kenalog or Depo-Medrol); 4 mL lidocaine; 22-gauge, 1½-inch needle
- Patient position: seated, arms at side
- Degree of difficulty: 6

The shoulder subacromial space injection is second only to the knee joint injection in terms of its importance and utility. Subacromial impingement is by far the most common condition you will see in adults with shoulder pain, and the subacromial injection plays a major role in nonoperative treatment of this frequently encountered diagnosis. The subacromial space can be injected from either a lateral or posterior approach. I favor the lateral approach, but the posterior approach also works well.

For the lateral approach, the patient is positioned sitting, with their arm at their side (Figure 9-10). Positioned in this way, the

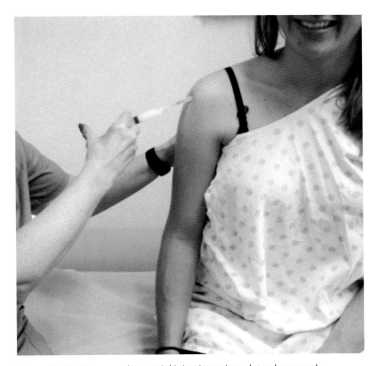

Figure 9-10. Giving a subacromial injection using a lateral approach.

weight of the arm helps pull the humerus down to open up the space. Start by identifying the posterior-lateral corner of the acromion (Figure 9-11). The scapular spine, a prominent bony ridge along the posterior aspect of the scapula, terminates as a bony process called the acromion. The scapular spine and the acromion look a little bit like the shaft and the blade of a hockey stick (Figure 9-12). The scapular spine and the posterior-lateral corner of the acromion are easy to palpate on even the heaviest patients.

To inject using a lateral approach, start at the posterior-lateral corner and move anteriorly, pressing hard with your finger to feel

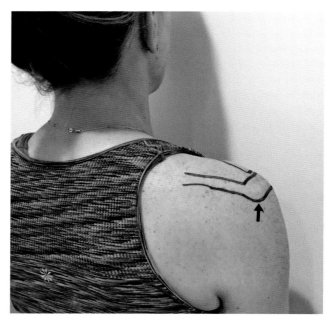

Figure 9-11. The posterior-lateral corner of the acromion (arrow) is a readily palpable bony prominence on the posterior aspect of the shoulder. It is the corner of the "hockey stick," where the scapular spine turns 90 degrees and becomes the acromion.

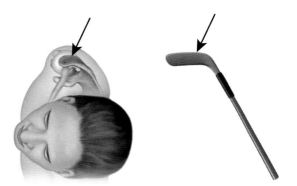

Figure 9-12. This drawing shows the location of the posterior-lateral corner of the acromion (arrow) and how the scapular spine and the acromion resemble the shaft and blade of a hockey stick.

the lateral edge of the acromion all the way to its tip (Figure 9-13). The lateral edge of the acromion is not as easy to palpate in obese or muscular patients. Pick a point about three-quarters of the way from the posterolateral corner to anterior tip of the lateral edge of the acromion (the white dot in Figure 9-13). The needle should enter 1-2 centimeters inferior to this point (at the *X* in Figure 9-14).

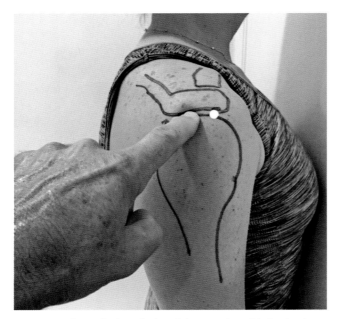

Figure 9-13. Defining the lateral edge of the acromion with the tip of your finger. The white dot indicates a point approximately three-quarters of the way from posterior to anterior.

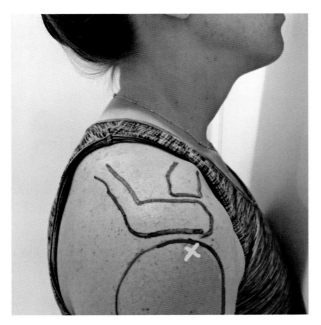

Figure 9-14. The ideal entry point for a subacromial space injection given using a lateral approach (marked with an *X*). The entry point should be three-quarters of the way from posterior to anterior and 1-2 centimeters *inferior to* the lateral edge of the acromion. Keep the entry point low. We want the needle to be angled from low to high when we give the injection.

Be sure your needle is not aiming parallel to the ground or aiming down. It should be aiming up at about a 45-degree angle (Figure 9-15). If you aim down or parallel to the ground, you may inadvertently inject the rotator cuff muscle or tendon rather than the subacromial space.

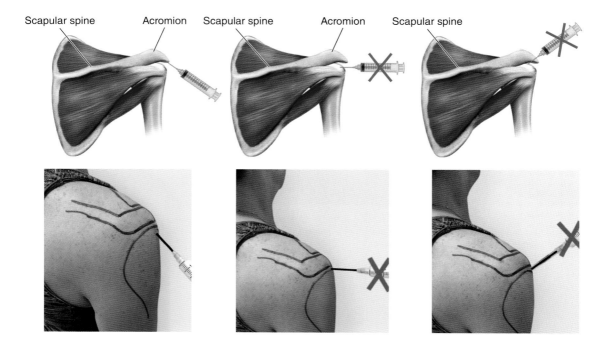

Figure 9-15. Direct the needle from inferior to superior (as depicted on the left image), not parallel to the ground or inferiorly (as depicted in the middle and right images, respectively).

After entering the skin, advance the needle (aiming superiorly) until the tip of the needle touches the edge of the acromion bone. (YES, we want to actually touch the edge of the acromion bone with the tip of the needle. This seems like it would hurt the patient, but it does not.) Once the needle has made contact with the lateral edge of the acromion, we want to "walk" the needle along the undersurface of the acromion and into the subacromial space. To do this, repeatedly advance the needle as you lower the angle of the needle inferiorly, millimeter by millimeter, until the needle advances along the undersurface of the acromion into the subacromial space (Figure 9-16).

If you prefer a posterior approach, start at the same starting point, the posterior-lateral corner of the acromion. Pick a point 1-2 centimeters medial and inferior to the posterolateral corner (Figure 9-17). The needle should enter here. Again, angle up,

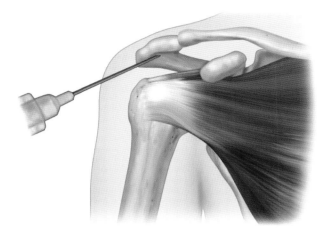

Figure 9-16. "Walking" the needle along the undersurface of the acromion bone. Slowly advance the needle as you lower the needle angle until you can feel the needle slide along the undersurface of the acromion.

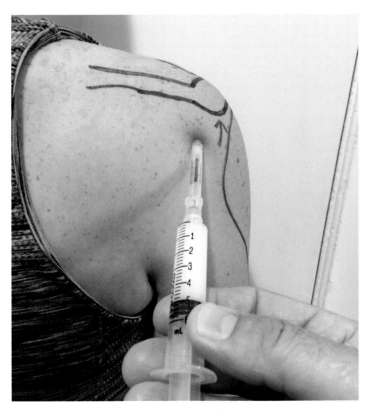

Figure 9-17. The entry point for a subacromial space injection using a posterior approach. The entry point is 1-2 centimeters inferior and medial to the posterior-lateral corner of the acromion (arrow).

not down or parallel to the ground. Advance the needle until it contacts the acromion bone, then walk under the acromion to enter the subacromial space.

If you are using a lateral approach, the needle should be inserted at least a centimeter deep to the point where contact was made with the lateral edge of the acromion before the injection is delivered. If you are using the posterior approach, you must go even deeper, at least 2 centimeters, before injecting. There should be little resistance as you inject the medication. If there is significant resistance, then the needle tip is not in the space, but in muscle, tendon, skin, or other connective tissue. Remove the needle and try again, confirming the landmarks before you start.

SHOULDER: Acromioclavicular (AC) Joint Injection

- **½ mL (20 mg) corticosteroid (Kenalog or Depo-Medrol); ½ mL lidocaine; 22-gauge, 1½-inch needle**
- **Patient position: seated, arms at side**
- **Degree of difficulty: 7**

This injection can be somewhat uncomfortable for patients because we are putting a relatively large volume of medicine into a relatively small space. Start by palpating the clavicle anywhere along its course from the sternum to the shoulder. The clavicle is a prominent subcutaneous structure and is easily palpable in even the heaviest patients. Once you have found the clavicle, move your finger laterally along its surface until you reach a bump or ridge on the superior surface of the very end of the clavicle (where it meets the acromion). Press hard with your fingernail to try to locate the 1- to 2-millimeter gap between the lateral end of the clavicle and the acromion (Figure 9-18). This gap is the AC joint space.

Prep the skin right over this gap. Orient the needle perpendicular to the skin and advance the needle. If the needle advances more than a few millimeters and doesn't hit bone, congratulations! You're in the AC joint! That's the equivalent of shooting a basketball through the hoop without it touching the rim! If you are like me, most of my shots don't "swoosh." I usually hit bone. If that's the case, pull back and reinsert a millimeter or two medially or laterally. Touching the bone with the needle like this does not hurt the patient. You may have to try several different points that are medial or lateral to your initial guess before you drop into the joint space, but when you do drop in, you will know it (Figure 9-19). The needle will drop in several millimeters instead of just hitting the bone directly beneath the skin.

Unlike injections into large, open spaces like the knee joint, glenohumeral joint, or subacromial space, you will encounter a fair amount of resistance as you inject into the AC joint because you are pushing a relatively large volume of medication into a relatively

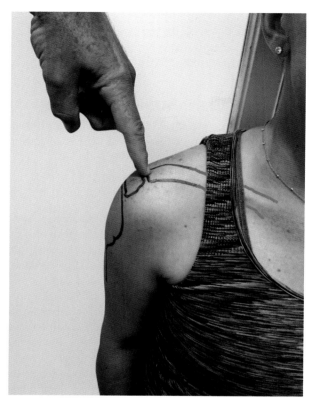

Figure 9-18. Feeling for the AC joint, which feels like a subtle gap between the end of the clavicle and the acromion. Pressing firmly with a fingernail can help you find the space.

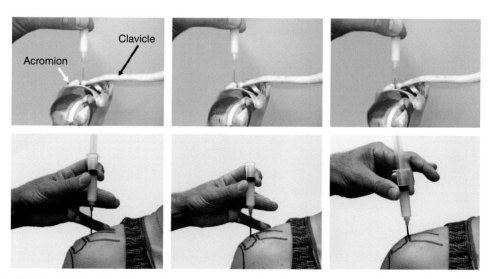

Figure 9-19. If you hit bone, try different spots before dropping into the AC joint. Keep the needle vertical. If you hit bone, pull out and try again a millimeter or two medially or laterally. When the needle drops into the space, you know you are in the joint.

small space. Do not advance the needle deeper than about a centimeter. If you do, the tip of the needle may pass through the AC joint and into the subacromial space beneath it, making the injection a subacromial space injection, not an AC joint injection.

SHOULDER: Glenohumeral Joint Injection

- 1 mL (40 mg) corticosteroid (Kenalog or Depo-Medrol); 4 mL lidocaine (Note: Unless the patient is very thin, you may need a 2-inch needle for this injection)
- Patient position: seated, arms at side
- Degree of difficulty: 7

To inject the glenohumeral joint, start by locating the posterolateral corner of the acromion (see the previous discussion in the section on subacromial space injections regarding how to locate the posterior-lateral corner of the acromion). The needle should enter the skin at a point 1-2 centimeters inferior and 1-2 centimeters medial to the posterior-lateral corner of the acromion. DO NOT AIM STRAIGHT ANTERIORLY! The surface of the glenoid socket is angled 45 degrees with respect to a line perpendicular to the coronal plane. This is important to understand when giving this injection. For a thorough explanation, review pages 70, and 76-77 in Chapter 2. Instead of aiming the needle anteriorly, aim 45 degrees toward the midline (Figure 9-20). The needle should advance a

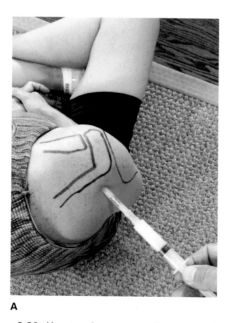
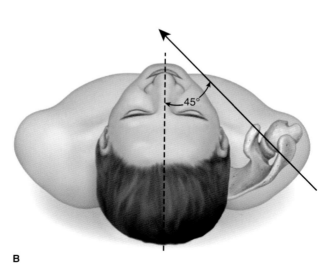

A   **B**

Figure 9-20. How to orient your needle to give a shoulder glenohumeral injection from a posterior approach. Remember to angle the needle 45 degrees toward the midline because the face of the glenoid is angled that way.

good 4 centimeters without touching bone, and the medication should inject without resistance.

As is the case with AC joint injections, unless you are very, very good or very, very lucky, you are likely to hit bone with your needle. This means that the needle tip is either hitting the scapula (medial to the joint space) or the humerus (lateral to the joint space). If you hit bone (and most likely you will), *don't panic!* You will be surprised to see that this does not hurt the patient, and we can use the information we learn from hitting the bone to redirect and enter the joint correctly.

Let me explain. If you advance the needle and hit bone, stop right there, but keep the needle where it is, on the surface of the bone you are hitting. Now, reach down and gently rotate the patient's humerus internally and externally (Figure 9-21). If your needle tip is pressed against the surface of the humerus, you will feel a grinding/grating as the humerus bone moves beneath the tip of the needle. If this is the case, you are too lateral and need to redirect medially. If the bone you are touching does not move as you rotate the humerus, then you are on the scapula and need to redirect laterally. Again, if you are in the right spot, you should be able to inject without much resistance.

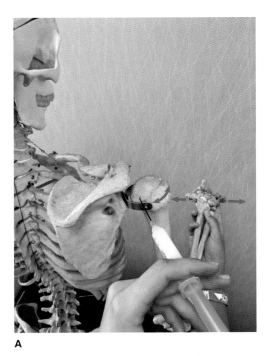 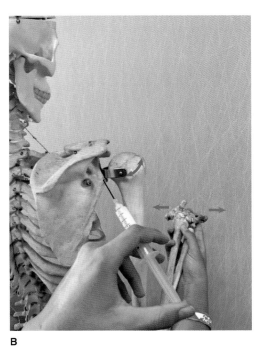

A   B

Figure 9-21. If you are performing a glenohumeral joint injection and hit bone, internally and externally rotate the humerus (by rotating the forearm) while the needle is on the bone. If you feel the bone move beneath your needle, you are on the humerus (left photo) and too lateral; redirect your needle more medially. If the bone you have hit does not move as you rotate the shoulder, you are on the scapula (right photo) and too medial. Redirect and move more laterally.

HIP: Greater Trochanteric Bursa Injection

- **1 mL of corticosteroid; 4 mL of lidocaine; 22-gauge, 1½-inch needle for thin patients or 22-gauge spinal needle for heavy patients**
- **Patient position: lying down lateral with affected side up**
- **Degree of difficulty: 1**

The cortisone injection for greater trochanteric bursitis is an easy injection to administer. Have the patient lie on their side, with the affected side up, and press firmly over the lateral side of the hip. You will find two firm, bony masses palpable beneath the skin. The higher one, approximately at the belt line, is the iliac crest (yellow arrow, Figure 9-22). The lower one (black arrow) is the greater trochanter. Use your fingers to find the place where the bone is closest to the skin. Prep this area and pick a point in the center of this area to enter with the needle. Orient your needle perpendicular to the ground and advance the needle *until you feel it contact the lateral surface of the femur bone*. This is very important. The medication must be delivered to the surface of the lateral femur. You must hit the bone with your needle. This will not hurt the patient. Expect a fair amount of tissue resistance as you inject. If the resistance is so high that you cannot get the medication to flow from the syringe, back off the surface of the bone a millimeter or two and you will find that the medication will flow easier.

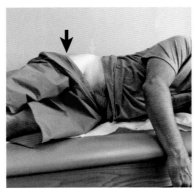
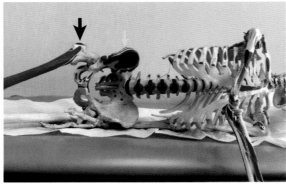

A   **B**

Figure 9-22. The location of the greater trochanter (black arrow). This bony feature is palpable with the patient in the lateral position on the exam table. This bony prominence is inferior to the iliac crest (yellow arrow).

HIP: Intra-Articular Hip Joint Injection

- **1 mL of corticosteroid; 4 mL of lidocaine; 22-gauge spinal needle**
- **NOTE: Requires image guidance; in this example, digital x-ray or fluoroscope**

- **Patient position: supine**
- **Degree of difficulty: 6**

Intra-articular cortisone injections can be helpful in the treatment of hip joint arthritis; the same injection technique can be used to aspirate the hip joint as part of a workup for gout or infection. The hip joint is deep enough below the surface of the skin that some method of image guidance is typically used to ensure that the needle is actually in the joint. Either ultrasound or x-ray imaging can work well for this procedure. We review a technique that uses an x-ray because it is the easiest to learn. If you don't have an x-ray or fluoroscope in your office, you can do this procedure in the x-ray department of your local hospital. Primary care residents whom I have trained who now work in rural communities will occasionally perform these injections. They are safe and simple.

The patient lies supine on the x-ray exam table, and the skin over the anterior groin is prepped. Center the x-ray beam over where you think the ball of the femoral head is (make your best guess), then lay the spinal needle on the skin so that its tip is directly over the femoral head (Figure 9-23). Again, make your best guess. Have the x-ray technician shoot a quick on/off "snapshot" single x-ray image. If you want to gown yourself with lead, you can stay by the patient's side. Otherwise, step a safe distance away from the patient when the x-ray is taken. Examine the image. Make necessary adjustments and reshoot the x-ray if needed to ensure that the femoral head is in the center of the image and the tip of the needle is lying over the center of the femoral head (approximately).

Once the patient, the x-ray beam, and the needle are positioned such that the center of the femoral head is in the center of the image and the tip of the needle is directly over the approximate

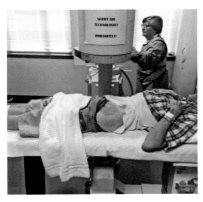 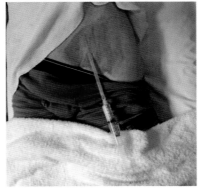 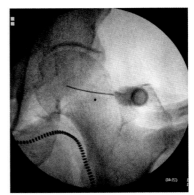

A   B   C

Figure 9-23. The technique for administering an x-ray–guided intra-articular hip joint injection (see text).

center of the femoral head, advance the needle through the skin until you hit bone. Take another image to ensure that the bone that the needle tip is touching is, indeed, the femoral head, and that the needle tip landed approximately on the center of the femoral head. Adjust the position of the needle as needed to ensure that this is the case.

Once the x-ray image has confirmed that the tip of the needle is resting right on the surface of the center of the femoral head and you feel the needle tip firmly on bone, try to inject. If you encounter significant resistance, back the tip of the needle off the surface of the bone 1-2 millimeters as you keep constant pressure on the plunger of the syringe. The tip of the needle may be embedded in the cartilage surface of the femoral head, and once the tip of the needle is out of the cartilage, the medication will flow freely. You do not need to inject contrast dye into the joint with this technique to confirm that you are in the joint. If the needle is touching the femoral head near its center, you are, by definition, in the joint.

It is quite possible that your needle will pass through the femoral artery, vein, or nerve on its path into the hip joint. A through-and-through puncture of any of these structures with a 22-gauge needle will not cause any serious harm. Injection of medication *into* the femoral artery, vein, or nerve could cause a serious complication, but these structures are far anterior to the surface of the femoral head, and a needle resting on the femoral head will not deliver an injection into these structures. If you do inadvertently puncture the artery or vein, hold firm pressure over the injection site for a full 5 minutes to prevent a possible hematoma.

HAND: Carpal Tunnel Injection

- **1 mL of corticosteroid; 1 mL of lidocaine; 22-gauge, 1½-inch needle**
- **Patient position: supine on the exam table with the arm outstretched, palm up**
- **Degree of difficulty: 5**

This injection is given on the palm side of the hand, through the skin and underlying transverse carpal ligament, and into the carpal tunnel. Start by identifying the transverse flexion creases (most of us have two) on the palmar side of the wrist. Pick a point in the midline 1-2 centimeters distal to the distal-most wrist crease (Figure 9-24). Prep and advance the needle perpendicular to the surface of the palm through the tough palmar skin. Once you have passed through the skin, advance the needle very slowly. The second you pass through the transverse carpal ligament (the dense roof of the carpal tunnel shown in the drawing on the right in Figure 9-24), the needle will likely touch the surface of the median nerve, which tends to lie in the midline.

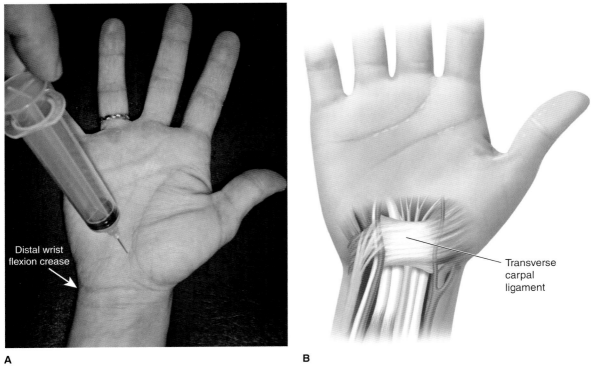

Figure 9-24. Most people have two wrist flexion creases. To find the stating point for a carpal tunnel injection, pick a point in the midline 1-2 centimeters distal to the most distal of the two wrist flexion creases.

As soon as the needle touches the median nerve, the patient will report a shooting pain or electrical sensation down the palm and into one or more of the fingers serviced by the median nerve (the thumb, index, middle, or lateral side of the ring finger). *Do not advance the needle any farther.* Instead, pull back very slowly until the patient reports that the pain or electrical sensation has gone away, then inject (Figure 9-25). Touching the median nerve with a 22-gauge needle will not damage it, but injecting into the substance of the nerve will. Be sure you don't inject until the shooting pain or electrical symptoms are gone.

If your patient's median nerve is not located in the midline or your injection entry point was slightly off center, the needle will keep advancing, and you won't hear anything about any shooting pain or electrical sensations. Eventually, the needle will hit one of the carpal bones that make up the floor of the carpal tunnel. If this happens, simply pull back off the bone surface a few millimeters and inject here. If your needle tip is hovering just over the surface of the floor of the carpal tunnel, you are in the carpal tunnel.

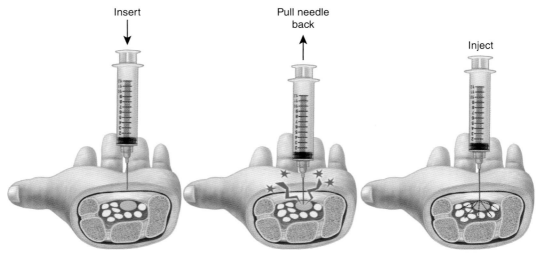

Figure 9-25. Advance the needle slowly once you pass beneath the skin (left drawing). The needle will most likely make contact with the median nerve, which will result in pain or an electrical sensation in the median nerve distribution (middle drawing). When this happens, pull the needle back just far enough to get its tip off the median nerve. You will know when the needle is off the nerve because the patient will no longer have the pain or electrical sensation. When this occurs, the needle is ideally positioned for the injection (right drawing).

Warn patients who receive carpal tunnel injections to expect increased numbness and tingling for a few hours after the injection because, if placed properly, the injection just delivered 1 mL of lidocaine directly onto the surface of the median nerve and will temporarily anesthetize it.

HAND: Trigger Finger Injection

- **½ mL (20 mg) corticosteroid (Kenalog or Depo-Medrol); ½ mL of lidocaine; 22-gauge, 1½-inch needle**
- **Patient position: supine on the exam table with the arm outstretched, palm up**
- **Degree of difficulty: 6**

To inject a trigger finger, first identify the metacarpal-phalangeal (MCP) joint crease at the base of the palm side of the finger to be injected (white arrow, Figure 9-26 B). Pick a point 1-2 centimeters proximal to the MCP crease *and exactly in the midline* of the affected finger. Advance the needle through the skin at an angle perpendicular to the surface of the palm. You will feel the needle enter the flexor tendon tissue, which is firm, dense, and rubbery. Gently apply pressure to the plunger on the syringe. Expect significant resistance because the needle tip is in the substance of the tendon.

Another way to confirm that the needle tip is in the substance of the tendon is to flex and extend the fingertip. If the needle rocks

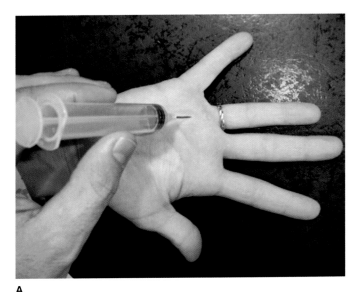

A

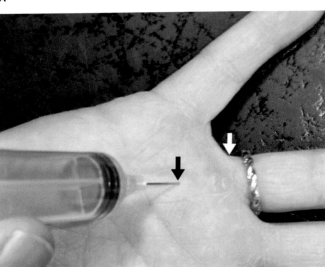

B

Figure 9-26. The entrance point for a trigger finger injection (black arrow) is in the midline of the affected finger, about 1-2 centimeters proximal to the metacarpal-phalangeal crease (white arrow).

back and forth, its tip is in the tendon. *Slowly* pull the needle back, keeping gentle pressure on the plunger. The instant the needle tip is pulled back out of the tendon, the medicine will flow freely (Figure 9-27).

The goal of this injection technique is *not to inject into the flexor tendon* (in fact, the flexor tendon can be damaged if the injection is given into it), but to inject into the tiny space between the surface

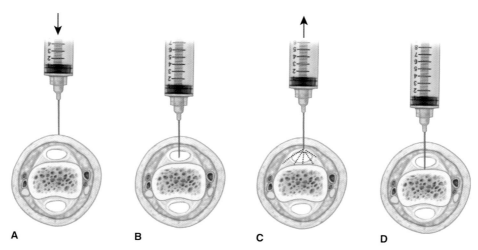

A   B   C   D

Figure 9-27. To administer a trigger finger injection, advance the needle slowly (**A**). Once you feel the needle enter the flexor tendon, which is dense and rubbery (**B**), gently press on the plunger of the syringe. You will encounter a lot of resistance. Maintain gentle pressure on the plunger of the syringe and pull back slowly on the needle. As soon as the needle tip pulls out of the tendon, the medicine will flow freely, and you will feel the loss of resistance (**C**). If you pull the needle back slowly enough, the tip of the needle will still be in the sheath of the tendon, which is the ideal location for this injection. If you pass through the tendon and hit the bone on the far side, you can deliver the injection here because the tendon sheath is immediately anterior to the bone (**D**).

of the tendon and the tendon sheath that surrounds it. Many times, you will feel or see the flexor tendon sheath of the finger "plump up" as the 1-milliliter volume of corticosteroid and lidocaine fill it. If the needle inadvertently passes all the way through the flexor tendon and exits the sheath on the back side, it will hit the anterior surface of the metacarpal bone just deep to the flexor tendon sheath. If this happens, pull back off the bone 1-millimeters and inject. Because the common digital nerve is near the flexor tendon sheath, patients receiving trigger finger injections may experience numbness in the injected digit for a few hours after the injection.

HAND: 1st Carpal-Metacarpal Joint (1st CMC Joint) Injection

- ½ mL (20 mg) corticosteroid (Kenalog or Depo-Medrol); ½ mL lidocaine; 22-gauge, 1½-inch needle
- Patient position: supine on the exam table with the arm outstretched, hand in neutral pronation/supination ("karate chop" position)
- Degree of difficulty: 6

This injection is given on the lateral side of the hand at the base of the thumb (Figure 9-28). The intended result is for the medication to be delivered into the 1st CMC joint, just proximal to the proximal end of the thumb metacarpal bone. To find the joint, find the thumb metacarpal bone, which resides just below the skin of the dorsal surface of the thumb. It is much harder to find the thumb

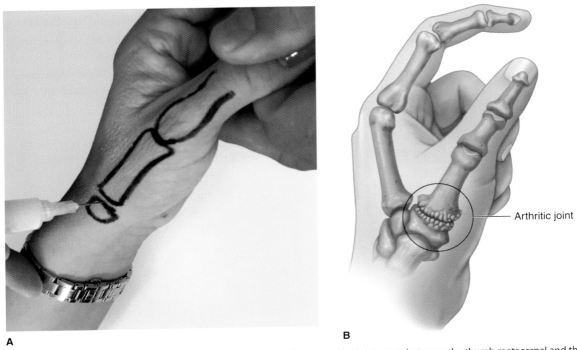

A   **B**

Arthritic joint

Figure 9-28. The injection site for the 1st CMC joint. The goal is to inject into the joint space between the thumb metacarpal and the trapezium. Pulling traction on the thumb will open the space.

metacarpal on the palm side of the hand because of the plump pad of muscles that make up the thenar eminence. For this reason, I recommend injecting on the dorsal side of the joint, where only a thin layer of skin lies between you and your target. Press hard with your fingernail on the skin over the dorsal surface of the thumb metacarpal as you move your finger from the midshaft of the metacarpal bone toward the proximal base. When you reach the proximal end of the bone, you will feel your fingernail drop into a subtle gap between the end of the thumb metacarpal bone and the trapezium bone just proximal to it. Sometimes rotating the thumb will help you identify where motion is occurring, that is, where the joint is. It also helps to pull longitudinal traction on the thumb. This will widen the 1st CMC joint space, giving you a better target.

Once you feel you have located the gap between the thumb metacarpal and the trapezium, try to pass the needle into that gap. If you fail and your needle hits bone, use the same strategy outlined in the previous section on AC joint injections: Repeat attempts more proximally or distally until you "fall into" the joint space, then inject. This injection hurts because we are instilling a large volume of medicine into a small space, and, as you depress the plunger on the syringe, you will encounter a fair amount of resistance for the same reason.

HAND: De Quervain Syndrome Injection

- ½ mL (20 mg) corticosteroid (Kenalog or Depo-Medrol); ½ mL lidocaine; 22-gauge, 1½-inch needle
- Patient position: supine on the exam table with the arm outstretched, hand in neutral pronation/supination ("karate chop" position)
- Degree of difficulty: 5

To perform this injection, we want to pass our needle into the sheath of the first extensor compartment (Figure 9-29).

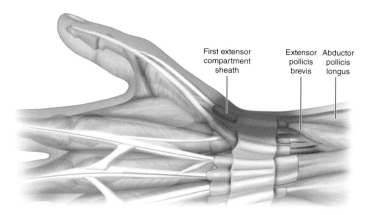

First extensor compartment sheath

Extensor pollicis brevis

Abductor pollicis longus

Figure 9-29. The anatomy of the dorsal side of the hand and wrist showing the extensor compartments. The tendons of the extensor pollicis brevis and abductor pollicis longus are in the first extensor compartment.

There are two tendons in this sheath: the extensor pollicis brevis and the abductor pollicis longus. The first extensor sheath makes up the lateral (closest to the thumb side of the wrist) border of the anatomic snuffbox (Figure 9-30). The sheath is usually palpable, and often visible where it crosses the wrist.

As is the case with the trigger finger injection (see previous discussion), we want our injection to be outside the substance of the tendon itself, but within the tendon sheath. To accomplish this, we will use the same technique used for the trigger finger injection. Prep, then enter the skin directly over the tendon sheath with the needle. Advance the needle until it enters the substance of the tendon, then apply gentle pressure to the plunger on the syringe. The medicine won't flow easily because the tendon tissue is too dense. As we draw the needle back slowly, there will be an instant when the medication suddenly flows without much resistance. That is the instant when the needle tip has left the substance of the tendon but is still within the tendon sheath. The sheath may "plump up" as the medication enters and distends it.

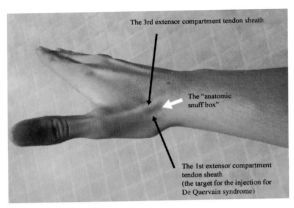

Figure 9-30. Use the anatomic snuffbox to locate the first extensor compartment. The injection for De Quervain syndrome is given into the first extensor compartment tendon sheath.

ELBOW: Medial and Lateral Epicondylitis Injection

- 1 mL (40 mg) corticosteroid (Kenalog or Depo-Medrol); 1 mL lidocaine; 22-gauge, 1½-inch needle
- Patient position: supine on the exam table, arm at side, elbow bent 90 degrees
- Degree of difficulty: 2

The key in administering an elbow epicondyle injection is correctly identifying the epicondyle (Figure 9-31). This is easiest with the elbow bent 90 degrees. It is easy to identify the olecranon process, the prominent posterior bony protuberance. The medial and lateral epicondyles are smaller, but still easy to palpate on all

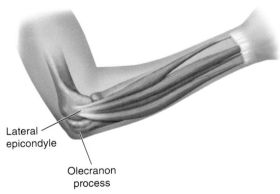

Figure 9-31. The lateral epicondyle of the distal humerus is the origin of the wrist and finger extensor muscles. The medial epicondyle is a similar bony prominence on the medial side of the elbow. It is the origin of the wrist and finger flexor muscles.

but the heaviest patients. Prep and inject directly over the epicondyle (Figure 9-32). Be sure your needle reaches and contacts the

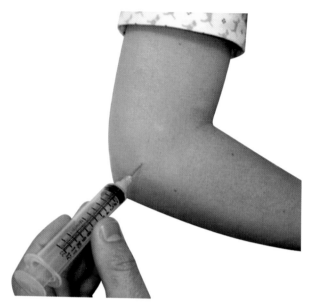

Figure 9-32. The injection for lateral epicondylitis is given directly onto the surface of the bony lateral epicondyle, a structure that is immediately beneath the skin and easily palpable on the lateral side of the elbow.

bone of the epicondyle. Many advocate moving the needle and injecting in multiple locations within a few millimeters of each other as the injection is given. This is an area where there is really only skin and bone, so expect the injection to leave a "bump."

Warning: Medial and lateral epicondyle injections have the highest risk of injection site complications, including 24-48 hours of severe injection site pain. Also, this injection is notorious for causing loss of pigmentation, fat atrophy, and a varicose-vein–like proliferation of the blood vessels in the skin at the injection site. These skin changes can show up months after the injection and may take months to resolve.

FOOT: Morton's Neuroma Injection

- 1 mL (40 mg) corticosteroid (Kenalog or Depo-Medrol); 1 mL lidocaine; 22-gauge, 1½-inch needle
- **Patient position: supine on exam table, knee and hip flexed so that the sole of the foot is flat on the table (Figure 9-33)**
- **Degree of difficulty: 3**

This injection is given between the metatarsal heads, just proximal to the webspace of the affected toes (Figure 9-34). It is

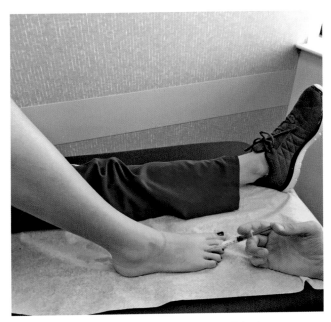

Figure 9-33. Patient position for a Morton's neuroma injection.

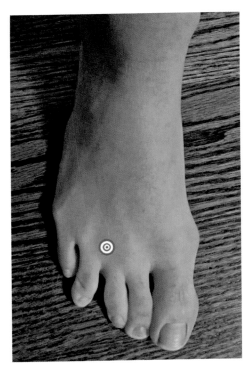

Figure 9-34. The location for a Morton's neuroma injection (target). The ideal place to inject is 1-2 centimeters proximal to the webspace of the affected toes on the dorsal surface of the foot.

best not to inject through the sole of the foot. Some of the corticosteroid could weep back through the injection tract and end up in the plantar fat on the sole of the foot, which could cause atrophy of this precious layer of padding that we rely on to walk comfortably. The needle should enter the skin on the dorsum of the foot 1-2 centimeters proximal to the webspace. Orient the needle perpendicular to the floor and insert the needle so that its tip is approximately halfway through the foot. There really isn't an open space here, so expect some resistance when you inject.

FOOT: Plantar Fascia Injection

- **1 mL corticosteroid; 1 mL lidocaine; 22-gauge, 1½-inch needle**
- **Patient position: supine on the exam table, affected foot hanging over the end of the table, contralateral hip and knee flexed (Figure 9-35)**

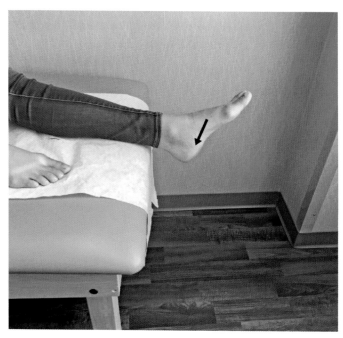

Figure 9-35. Patient position for a plantar fascia injection.

As mentioned, we try to avoid injecting through the fat pad on the plantar surface of the foot. The target we are trying to hit is the place on the anterior edge of the plantar surface of the calcaneus where the plantar fascia inserts (Figure 9-36). We can reach this target through a medial approach. To start, palpate the anterior edge of the calcaneus. Prep the skin and pick an entry point and trajectory that will allow your needle to reach the anterior

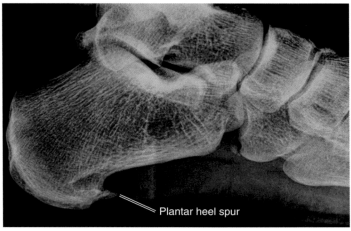

Plantar heel spur

A

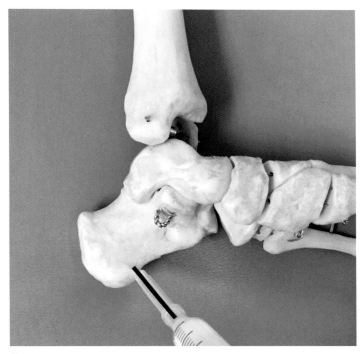

B

Figure 9-36. The target for the plantar fascia injection is the origin of the plantar fascia on the anterior calcaneus, the same place the bone spur tends to be in patients with plantar fasciitis.

edge of the calcaneus bone (Figure 9-37). Advance the needle until you feel it touch the bone. Walk the needle tip anteriorly along the calcaneus until it falls off the front edge and you don't feel it hitting bone any longer. Then, move back to where you are hitting bone again. This ensures that you are on the anterior edge of

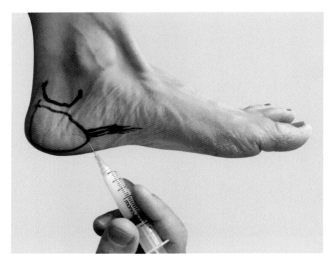

Figure 9-37. The entry point for a plantar fascia injection. Find the medial edge of the calcaneus by pressing hard against the medial heel with your finger. Try to feel where the bone ends. Aim for that point, at the very front of the plantar surface of the calcaneus.

the calcaneus. Inject here. Expect resistance, as this tissue is very dense. *It is also richly innervated, so this injection is typically very painful.*

ANKLE: Ankle Joint Injection

- **1 mL (40 mg) corticosteroid (Kenalog or Depo-Medrol); 1 mL lidocaine; 22-gauge, 1½-inch needle**
- **Patient position: supine on exam table, knee and hip flexed and foot flat on the table (same as Morton's neuroma injection position [see Figure 9-33]).**
- **Degree of difficulty: 7**

It is safest to enter the ankle joint from an anterior-lateral approach. The landmarks are the tip of the fibula and the anterior edge of the talus (Figure 9-38). The tip of the fibula is easily palpated on the lateral side of the ankle, but the anterior edge of the talus is more difficult to identify. Flexing the ankle joint up and down while applying firm pressure with your fingers over the anterior ankle can help you determine where the joint is by feeling for which bone is moving (the talus) and which bone isn't (the tibia). Prep the skin and pick a point 1 centimeter anterior to the anterior edge of the fibula at the level of the joint line. Aim posteriorly and medially. If you hit bone, keep your needle tip on the bone that you've hit and flex the ankle up and down. You will be able to feel whether the bone beneath the needle is moving or not. If it is moving, you are on the talus, and you need to try again more superiorly. If the bone is not moving, you are on the tibia,

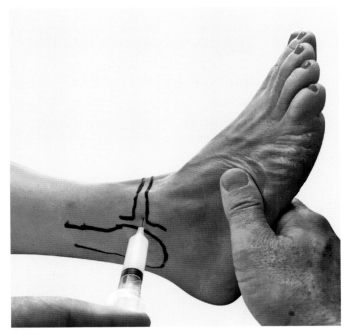

A

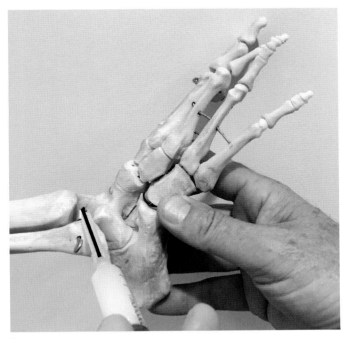

B

Figure 9-38. The point of entry for an ankle joint injection. The needle should enter the skin 1 centimeter medial to the medial edge of the fibula (lateral malleolus) at the level of the joint line. The joint line can be hard to find. Flex the ankle up and down and try to determine where the motion is occurring. That is the joint line.

and you need to try again more inferiorly. If you are in the right spot, you will drop into the joint space a good centimeter, and there will be very little resistance when you inject.

SPINE: Caudal Epidural Steroid Injection

- **1 mL corticosteroid; *5 mL sterile NaCl (NOT lidocaine)*; 22-gauge, 1½-inch needle**
- **Patient position: prone on the exam table**
- **Degree of difficulty: 6**

The technique for administering an in-office lumbar epidural steroid injection takes advantage of an anatomic feature known as the sacral hiatus (Figure 9-39). It is a small opening at the base

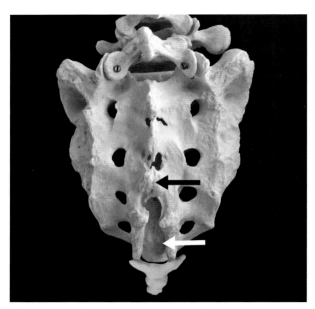

Figure 9-39. The sacral hiatus (white arrow) is an opening in the bony tunnel that surrounds the spinal canal at the lower end of the sacrum. It allows safe access to the epidural space of the lumbosacral spine. The black arrow points to a part of the sacrum that is covered with thick, dense bone. If you are administering a caudal epidural and your needle hits bone and won't advance, you are likely on an area like this. Move up or down, staying in the midline, until you find the opening.

of the sacrum just above the coccyx that allows us to enter the lumbar epidural space. Because corticosteroids are soluble in fat and the epidural space is full of fat, the medication readily diffuses up the epidural space and can reach the lower lumbar spine. I recommend you use normal saline instead of lidocaine for this injection because lidocaine injected into the epidural space can result in an *epidural anesthetic*, causing temporary motor and sensory dysfunction. This injection may not be as useful for pathology in the upper lumbar spine, but most lumbar pathology is below the level of the fourth lumbar vertebra. This technique is sometimes referred to as a "poor man's epidural" because it is not injected directly at the site of the lumbar pathology under image guidance. It is not as effective as lumbar epidural injection given that way. The advantage is that it is safe and simple and can be given in an office setting.

At the level of the bottom of the sacrum, where this injection is given, all of the nerve roots have exited the spinal canal. There are no nerve roots to injure, no dural sleeves to puncture, and a hematoma at this location will not create a mass effect on adjacent neural tissue (because there is no neural tissue here). Although it has not been proven particularly effective for treating low back pain, the caudal epidural steroid injection has been shown to help patients with radicular symptoms and can be an important tool for conservative management of patients with lumbosacral radiculopathy.

To administer the injection, carefully prep the skin just above the intergluteal fold. The opening is in the midline, and it is narrow. Pick a point exactly in the midline 2-3 centimeters above (superior to) the top of the intergluteal fold (Figure 9-40). Enter here with your needle with the needle angled superiorly toward the patient's

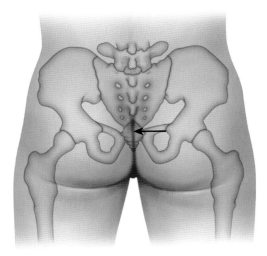

Figure 9-40. The location of the entry point for a caudal epidural is in the midline, just above the top of the intergluteal fold (also known as the "butt crack").

head. Press firmly and feel for a "pop" as the needle passes through the layer of dense, tough fibrous tissue that is stretched like a sheet over the opening of the sacral hiatus. In many instances, this layer of fibrous tissue is partially calcified and passing a needle through it will feel a little crunchy, like passing a needle through an eggshell.

If you are pressing firmly and the needle feels like it is on solid bone and it simply won't advance, you may have landed on a place where there is a thick layer of bone. If that is the case, try again through a different site superior or inferior to the spot you just tried, but always stay exactly in the midline. The sacral hiatus is variable in its length from superior to inferior, but it is always in the midline. It is common to have to try this injection several times through several spots before finding the opening. Once you do find the spot, you will feel the "pop" as described previously, then the needle will "drop" through the canal of the epidural space and then "stop" as it hits the bony floor of the spinal canal (Figure 9-41).

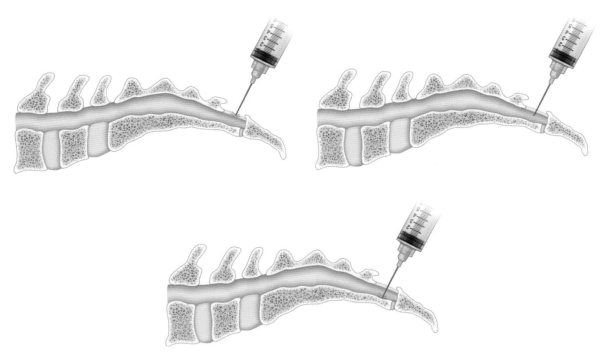

Figure 9-41. A lateral view of the sacrum. When you successfully inject through the sacral hiatus, you feel a "pop" (drawing on the top left) as the needle passes through a tough, dense membrane of fibrous tissue, then a "drop" (drawing on the top right) as the needle falls through the spinal canal, and finally a "stop" (drawing on the bottom) as the needle hits the back wall of the epidural space.

If you are in the right place, there is almost no resistance as you inject. If there is a lot of resistance, you are in the wrong place, and you need to start over. Another sure sign that you have not successfully penetrated into the epidural space and are injecting onto the surface of the sacrum is the appearance of a growing mound of soft tissue swelling as you inject. The swelling results from the medication infiltrating the skin over the surface of the sacrum, which, at this location, is essentially subcutaneous.

Index

Page numbers followed by *f* or *t* indicate figures or tables, respectively.